Dear Reader

I'm Lia Levicky, and I'm thrilled to have you join my journey. Thank you for picking up this book—I hope it brings you joy and inspiration. Let's embark on this adventure together!

The "Discovering the Blue Zone Diet Cookbook for Two" is a delightful journey through flavors where I've gathered and detailed 95 recipes. Choosing this particular number wasn't a random decision.

Imagine uncovering the secret to a long, vibrant life inspired by a deeply personal story. My journey into the realm of Blue Zones and the quest for longevity began with the awe-inspiring lives of my own grandmother and her identical twin sister. My grandmother lived a remarkable life, passing away at the age of 92, while her identical twin sister reached an impressive age of 95. Their longevity inspired me to reflect on what I could do to improve my own chances of reaching 90 and beyond.

This fascination led me to explore the world of Blue Zones, regions where people seem to have found the fountain of youth. What captivated me was the revelation that these remarkable lifespans were not solely the result of genetics, but the profound impact of lifestyle choices. It's a journey that reveals the importance of nutrition, the magic of wholesome foods, and the enchantment of connecting with nature.

Embarking on this exciting journey, I've come to realize that we each possess the power to craft our destinies, unveiling the secrets to a longer, healthier life.

I'm excited to share the enchanting discoveries, and I hope to inspire others to join me on this mesmerizing journey toward greater well-being and longevity.

SNACKS AND APPETIZERS FOR VITALITY

- AVOCADO AND BLACK BEAN SALSA...5
- WATERMELON AND FETA SKEWERS...5
- DATE AND NUT ENERGY BITES...6
- WALNUT-STUFFED DATES...6
- ALMOND DATE BALLS...7
- CHIA SEED PUDDING...7
- HUMMUS MEZZE PLATTE..8
- BLUEBERRY OATMEAL BARS..8
- CLASSIC HUMMUS..9
- MEDITERRANEAN HERB AND OLIVE HUMMUS...............................10
- EGGPLANT AND TOMATO BRUSCHETTA...11
- DATE AND NUT STUFFED BAKED APPLES......................................12
- BANANA WALNUT MUFFINS..13
- ALMOND AND HONEY RICE PUDDING..14

WHOLESOME SOUPS

- LENTIL AND VEGETABLE SOUP..15
- KALE AND WHITE BEAN SOUP...16
- BARLEY AND MUSHROOM SOUP...17
- SPINACH AND CHICKPEA SOUP..18
- CABBAGE AND POTATO SOUP..19
- TOMATO LENTIL SOUP...20
- SWEET POTATO AND GINGER SOUP..21
- QUINOA AND VEGETABLE SOUP...22
- TURMERIC AND CAULIFLOWER SOUPS...23
- GREEN PEA AND MINT SOUP..24
- VEGAN MISO SOUP...25
- MISO SOUP WITH TOFU AND SEAWEED.......................................26
- MINESTRONE SOUP..27

SATISFYING SALADS AND FLAVOURED BREAD FOR LONGEVITY

- MEDITERRANEAN CHICKPEA SALAD..28
- TZATZIKI CUCUMBER SALAD..28
- OKINAWAN SEARED AHI TUNA SALAD..29
- CUCUMBER CUPS WITH TUNA SALAD..30
- CAPRESE SALAD...30

MEDITERRANEAN TABBOULEH SALAD	31
OKINAWAN TOFU AND SEAWEED SALAD	32
CABBAGE AND CARROT SLAW	32
TASTY SALAD WITH GRILLED CHICKEN	33
MEDITERRANEAN WHOLE GRAIN BREAD	34
SARDINIAN PANE CARASAU (FLATBREAD)	35
OKINAWAN SWEET POTATO BREAD	36
DELICIOUS WHOLE WHEAT PITA BREAD	36
REGIONAL MOCHI BREAD	37

SIDE DISHES THAT NOURISH

ROASTED ASPARAGUS WITH LEMON AND PARMESAN	38
SWEET POTATO AND CHICKPEA PATTIES	39
MEDITERRANEAN ROASTED EGGPLANT	40
LENTIL AND VEGETABLE STEW	40
WHOLESOME TZATZIKI AND VEGGIE PLATTER	41
ROASTED BEET AND GOAT CHEESE CROSTINI	41
ROASTED RED PEPPER AND WALNUT DIP	42
SPINACH AND FETA STUFFED MINI PEPPERS	43
STUFFED MUSHROOMS WITH QUINOA AND SPINACH	43
SUNNY CAPRESE STUFFED PORTOBELLO MUSHROOMS	44
QUINOA AND BLACK BEAN STUFFED PEPPERS	45

DELECTABLE MAIN COURSES FOR HEALTH

VEGAN TAGINE WITH CHICKPEAS	46
OKINAWAN STIR-FRIED VEGETABLES	47
FLAVORFUL LEMON AND GARLIC ROASTED CHICKEN	47
GRILLED CHICKEN WITH HERBED QUINOA	48
OSSO BUCO (VEAL OR BEEF SHANK STEW)	49
ROASTED GARLIC AND WHITE BEAN DIP	50
QUINOA-STUFFED BELL PEPPERS	51
ZUCCHINI AND TOMATO SKEWERS	51
TOFU AND VEGETABLE STIR-FRY	52
GRILLED EGGPLANT AND ZUCCHINI RATATOUILLE	53
WHOLE WHEAT PASTA PRIMAVERA	53
BROWN RICE AND BLACK BEAN BOWL	54
SAUTÉED GREENS WITH WHITE BEANS	54

SEAFOOD SPECIALS FOR WELLNESS

- BAKED SALMON WITH LEMON AND DILL..................55
- BAKED HALIBUT WITH TOMATOES AND OLIVES..............55
- GRILLED OCTOPUS..................56
- OKINAWAN SEARED TUNA STEAK..................56
- VIBRANT SUSHI BOWLS..................57
- SARDINIAN FREGOLA WITH CLAMS..................57
- GRILLED WHOLE SEA BASS..................58
- EASY TERIYAKI SALMON..................58
- EXOTIC MISO-GLAZED SALMON..................59

GLOBAL FLAVORS AND LONGEVITY

- FALAFEL WITH HUMMUS AND BULGUR SALAD..................60
- MEDITERRANEAN STUFFED GRAPE LEAVES..................61
- CAPRESE SKEWERS..................62
- OKINAWAN BRAISED PORK BELLY..................62
- SARDINIAN LAMB AND ARTICHOKE STEW..................63
- BIFTEKIA (GRILLED MEAT PATTIES)..................64
- EGGPLANT AND WALNUT ROLLS..................64
- SPANAKOPITA (SPINACH PIE)..................65
- MEDITERRANEAN BAKED EGGPLANT PARMESAN..................66
- EGGPLANT AND ZUCCHINI RATATOUILLE..................67

SWEETS TO SAVOR WITHOUT GUILT

- BAKED APPLES WITH CINNAMON..................68
- FIG AND WALNUT BARS..................69
- LEMON SORBET..................69
- PEACH AND BERRY COBBLER..................70
- BERRY AND YOGURT PARFAIT..................70
- ORANGE AND DATE SALAD..................71
- COCONUT CHIA PUDDING..................71
- OATMEAL RAISIN COOKIES..................72
- BANANA "NICE" CREAM..................72
- ROASTED FRUIT SALAD..................73
- PAPAYA WITH LIME..................73

ALPHABETICAL RECIPE INDEX....74

AVOCADO AND BLACK BEAN SALSA

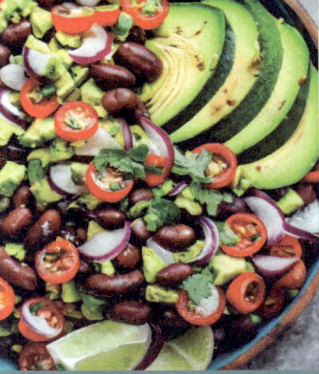

COOKING PROCESS:

Begin by dicing the ripe avocados and placing them in a mixing bowl. Drain and rinse the black beans thoroughly, then add them to the bowl with the avocados. If using frozen corn, thaw it by briefly microwaving or cooking it according to the package instructions. If using canned or fresh corn, make sure it's cooked and cooled before adding it to the mixture. Quarter the cherry tomatoes, finely chop the red onion and chop the fresh cilantro leaves.
In the mixing bowl with the avocados and black beans, add the corn kernels, quartered cherry tomatoes, finely chopped red onion, and chopped cilantro.
In a separate small bowl, prepare the dressing by whisking together the juice of limes, extra virgin olive oil, minced garlic, and salt and pepper to taste.
Drizzle the dressing over the avocado and black bean mixture. Gently toss all the ingredients together until they are well coated with the dressing.
Refrigerate the Avocado and Black Bean Salsa for about 30 minutes before serving. This allows the flavors to meld together and enhances the freshness.
Once chilled, transfer the salsa to a serving bowl or dish. Serve the salsa with tortilla chips for scooping and enjoying.

INGREDIENTS:

- 2 ripe avocados
- 1 can (15 ounces) of black beans
- 1 cup corn kernels (frozen or fresh)
- 1 cup cherry tomatoes
- 1/2 red onion
- 1/4 cup fresh cilantro Juice of 2 limes
- 2 tablespoons extra virgin olive oil
- 1-2 cloves garlic
- Salt and pepper, to taste
- Tortilla chips (for serving)

WATERMELON AND FETA SKEWERS

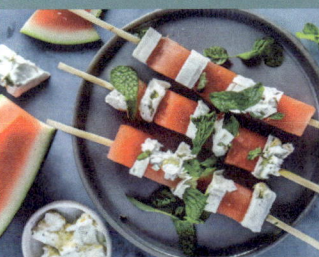

Slice the watermelon into approximately 1-inch thick rounds. You can remove the rind if desired for easier handling. Use a small round cookie cutter or a knife to cut out bite-sized watermelon rounds.
Cut the feta cheese into small cubes that are roughly the same size as the watermelon rounds.
Take a wooden skewer or cocktail toothpick and first thread on a watermelon round. Follow with a cube of feta cheese and a fresh mint leaf. Continue this pattern until the skewer is filled, leaving a small portion at the top for easy handling. Repeat this process for as many skewers as you'd like to prepare.
Drizzle a bit of balsamic glaze over the skewers for a sweet and tangy flavor. Arrange the watermelon and feta skewers on a serving platter.

- 1 small seedless watermelon
- 8 ounces feta cheese
- 1 bunch fresh mint leaves
- 1/4 cup balsamic reduction or balsamic glaze (store-bought or homemade)
- Wooden skewers or cocktail toothpicks

Snacks and Appetizers for Vitality

DATE AND NUT ENERGY BITES

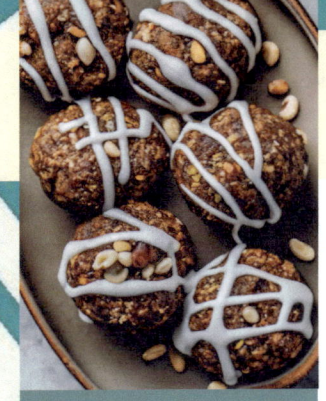

INGREDIENTS:
- 1 cup pitted dates
- 1/2 cup almonds
- 1/2 cup walnuts
- 1/4 cup rolled oats
- 1 tablespoon chia seeds (optional)
- 1 teaspoon vanilla extract (optional)
- A pinch of salt (optional)
- Desiccated coconut or cocoa powder for rolling (optional)

COOKING PROCESS:

Start by placing 1 cup of pitted dates into a food processor. If the dates are very dry, you can soak them in warm water for a few minutes to soften them before using.

Add to the food processor almonds, walnuts, rolled oats, chia seeds (if desired for added nutrition), vanilla extract (for flavor, if desired) and a pinch of salt (if desired). Pulse the ingredients in the food processor until they are finely chopped and the mixture starts to come together. You should have a sticky, dough-like consistency.

Stop the food processor and scrape down the sides if needed to ensure all ingredients are evenly mixed.

Once the mixture is ready, scoop out small portions and roll them into bite-sized balls with your hands. You can make them as large or small as you like.

If desired, roll the energy bites in desiccated coconut or cocoa powder for an extra layer of flavor and texture.

Place the rolled energy bites on a plate or tray and refrigerate them for at least 30 minutes to firm up.

After chilling, your Date and Nut Energy Bites are ready to enjoy! You can store them in an airtight container in the refrigerator for several days.

WALNUT-STUFFED DATES

- 16 large Medjool dates
- 16 walnut halves
- A pinch of sea salt (optional)
- Ground cinnamon for dusting (optional)

Take dates and using a small knife, make a lengthwise slit in each date to create an opening. Be careful not to cut the date in half completely; you want to create a pocket for the walnut.

Take walnut halves and insert one walnut half into each date, placing it where you made the slit. The combination of sweet dates and crunchy walnuts is a delightful contrast.

If you like, you can add a pinch of sea salt to each stuffed date. The salt enhances the flavors by balancing the sweetness of the dates and the nuttiness of the walnuts.

Optionally, you can also dust the stuffed dates with a bit of ground cinnamon for added flavor and aroma.

Arrange the Walnut-Stuffed Dates on a serving platter or plate.

These stuffed dates can be enjoyed immediately as a quick and healthy dessert or snack. They are naturally sweet and satisfying.

ALMOND DATE BALLS

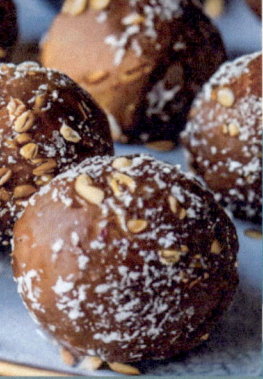

COOKING PROCESS:

Begin by placing pitted dates in a food processor. If your dates are very dry, you can soak them in warm water for about 10 minutes to soften them before processing. Add almonds to the food processor with the dates. You can use raw almonds or lightly toasted almonds for added flavor.

If you'd like to enhance the flavor, add 1 teaspoon of vanilla extract and a pinch of salt. Pulse the ingredients in the food processor until they start to come together into a sticky, dough-like consistency.

Add an unsweetened shredded coconut into the mixture at this stage. Pulse until it's well combined with the other ingredients. Once the mixture is ready, it should be sticky enough to hold together when you press it between your fingers.

Form the almond date balls. You can adjust the size to your preference. You can roll the almond date balls in additional shredded coconut or crushed almonds to add a coating for extra texture and flavor.

Place the formed balls on a tray or plate lined with parchment paper. Refrigerate for at least 30 minutes to allow them to firm up and hold their shape.

Once they have chilled, your Almond Date Balls are ready to enjoy.

INGREDIENTS:
- 1 cup almonds
- 1 cup pitted dates
- 1/4 cup unsweetened shredded coconut
- 1/4 teaspoon cinnamon
- A pinch of salt (optional)
- Additional shredded coconut or crushed almonds for coating (optional)

CHIA SEED PUDDING

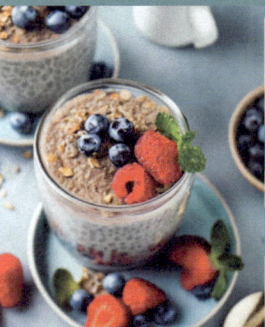

In a mixing bowl, combine chia seeds, and unsweetened almond milk (or your preferred milk). If you like your Chia Seed Pudding sweet, add 2-4 tablespoons of honey or maple syrup (adjust to your desired level of sweetness). You can also add 1 teaspoon of vanilla extract for extra flavor. Stir well to combine all the ingredients.

Once the mixture is well combined, cover the bowl and refrigerate it for at least 4 hours or overnight. This allows the chia seeds to absorb the liquid and create a pudding-like texture.

After the resting period, give the Chia Seed Pudding a good stir to redistribute the seeds. You'll notice that the mixture has thickened considerably.

To serve, spoon the Chia Seed Pudding into individual serving dishes or glasses.

Top the pudding with fresh fruit or berries of your choice: strawberries, blueberries, or banana slices work wonderfully. For added texture and nutrition, garnish with chopped nuts (almonds, walnuts) or sunflower seeds.

Feel free to get creative with your toppings based on your preferences.

- 1/2 cup chia seeds
- 2 cups unsweetened almond milk
- 2-4 tablespoons honey or maple syrup
- 1 teaspoon vanilla extract (optional)
- Fresh fruit or berries for topping
- Nuts or seeds for garnish

Snacks and Appetizers for Vitality

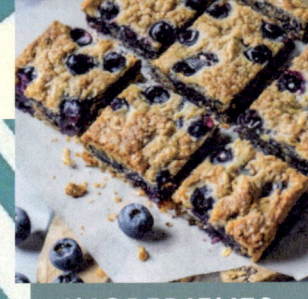

BLUEBERRY OATMEAL BARS

INGREDIENTS:

- 2 cups rolled oats
- 1 cup whole wheat flour
- 1/2 cup honey
- 1/4 cup unsweetened applesauce
- 1 cup fresh or frozen blueberries
- 1/2 tsp cinnamon
- 1/4 teaspoon salt

COOKING PROCESS:

Preheat the oven to 350°F (175°C) and grease an 8x8-inch baking dish. In a large mixing bowl, combine: rolled oats, whole wheat flour, cinnamon, and salt.

In a separate bowl, mix the wet ingredients: honey and unsweetened applesauce. Pour the wet mixture over the dry ingredients and stir until well combined. The mixture should resemble a crumbly texture.

Take half of the crumbly mixture and press it evenly into the bottom of the prepared baking dish. This forms the bottom crust. Spread fresh or frozen blueberries evenly over the crust. Sprinkle the remaining crumbly mixture over the blueberries. Gently press it down with a spatula.

Bake in the preheated oven for 30-35 minutes, or until the top is golden brown and the blueberries are bubbling. Remove from the oven and let it cool in the baking dish for about 10-15 minutes.

After cooling slightly, carefully lift the entire slab out of the baking dish using the parchment paper as handles. Place it on a wire rack to cool completely.

Once the Bars are completely cooled, cut them into squares or rectangles. Serve and enjoy these delicious and nutritious oatmeal bars with a blueberry twist.

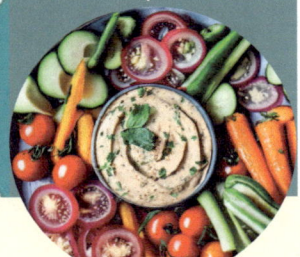

HUMMUS MEZZE PLATTE

FOR THE HUMMUS:
- 1 can (15 ounces) of chickpeas (garbanzo beans)
- 2-3 tbsp of tahini (sesame paste)
- 2-3 cloves of garlic
- 1 lemon
- 2-3 tbsp of extra virgin olive oil
- Salt and pepper
- Water

FOR THE PLATTER:
- Fresh vegetables (such as cucumber slices, cherry tomatoes, baby carrots, bell peppe strips)
- Kalamata olives
- Feta cheese
- Fresh parsley or mint eaves
- Whole-grain pita bread or pita chips

In a food processor, combine the drained and rinsed chickpeas, tahini, minced garlic, juice of lemon, and oil.

Season with salt and pepper to taste. Blend the ingredients until you achieve a smooth and creamy consistency. If the hummus is too thick, you can add a bit of water (1-2 tbsp at a time) and blend until it reaches your desired texture.

Taste the hummus and adjust the seasonings if necessary. You can add more lemon juice, garlic, or salt based on your preference.

Arrange the freshly prepared hummus in a shallow serving dish or on a platter, creating a well in the center with the back of a spoon.

Surround the hummus with an array of fresh vegetables. Sprinkle Kalamata olives and crumbled feta cheese over the hummus for added flavor and texture. Garnish the platter with fresh parsley or mint leaves for a touch of greenery.

Hummus is best enjoyed fresh. Serve it with warm pita bread or pita chips alongside the platter to scoop up the hummus and enjoy the fresh vegetables or as a spread in sandwiches and wraps.

Snacks and Appetizers for Vitality

CLASSIC HUMMUS

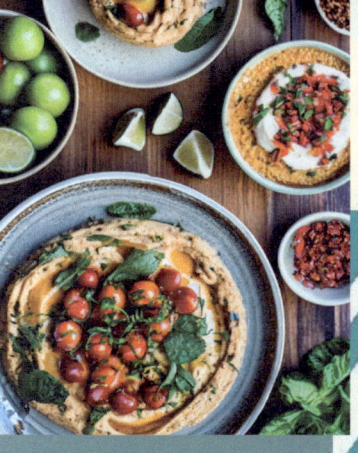

COOKING PROCESS:

Start by opening a can of chickpeas (garbanzo beans). Drain them in a colander and rinse thoroughly under cold running water. Rinsing helps remove excess salt and starch, resulting in smoother hummus.

Gather your ingredients: chickpeas, fresh lemon juice, tahini (sesame paste), minced garlic, extra-virgin olive oil, ground cumin, salt, water, ground paprika (optional for garnish), and fresh parsley (optional for garnish).

In a food processor, add the drained and rinsed chickpeas, fresh lemon juice, well-stirred tahini, minced garlic, extra-virgin olive oil, ground cumin, and a pinch of salt.

Turn on the food processor and let it run for about 2-3 minutes. During this time, the ingredients will start to break down and blend together. You might need to scrape down the sides of the processor with a spatula to ensure everything gets mixed evenly.

With the food processor running, add 2 to 3 tablespoons of water gradually through the feed tube. This will help achieve the creamy and smooth texture you desire. Continue processing for a couple more minutes until the hummus is velvety.

Turn off the food processor and give your hummus a taste. At this point, you can adjust the seasoning to your preference. If you want more lemony flavor, add extra lemon juice. Adjust the salt to taste.

Scoop the freshly made hummus into a serving bowl. Using the back of a spoon, create a shallow well or swirl pattern in the center of the hummus.

Drizzle a generous splash of extra-virgin olive oil into the well or over the surface of the hummus. This adds richness and a lovely sheen. Optionally, sprinkle a dash of ground paprika for a touch of color and flavor. You can also add some chopped fresh parsley for freshness and presentation.

INGREDIENTS:

- 1 can (15 ounces) chickpeas (garbanzo beans)
- 1/4 cup fresh lemon juice (1 large lemon)
- 1/4 cup well-stirred tahini (sesame paste)
- 1 small garlic clove
- 2 tablespoons extra-virgin olive oil, plus more, for serving
- 1/2 teaspoon ground cumin
- Salt to taste
- 2 to 3 tablespoons water
- Dash of ground paprika, for garnish (optional)
- Fresh parsley, for garnish (optional)

Snacks and Appetizers for Vitality

MEDITERRANEAN HERB AND OLIVE HUMMUS

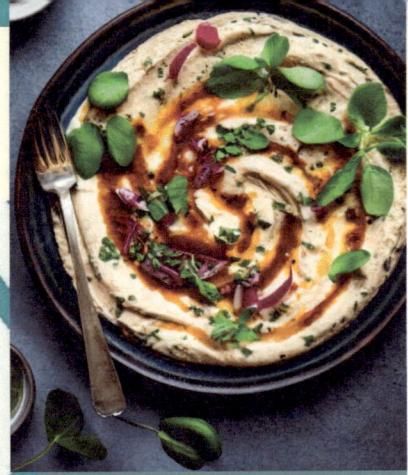

INGREDIENTS:

- 2 cups cooked chickpeas (canned or freshly cooked)
- 1/4 cup fresh lemon juice (about 2 lemons)
- 1/4 cup tahini
- 2 cloves garlic
- 1/4 cup extra virgin olive oil, plus more for serving
- 1/2 teaspoon ground cumin
- 1/2 teaspoon paprika, plus more for garnish
- 1/2 teaspoon salt, or to taste
- 1/4 teaspoon freshly ground black pepper, or to taste
- 1/2 cup fresh herbs (such as parsley, cilantro, or a mix)
- 1/2 cup Kalamata olives

COOKING PROCESS:

If you're using canned chickpeas, start by rinsing them thoroughly in a colander under cold running water. Drain well. If you're using freshly cooked chickpeas, ensure they are well-drained.

In the bowl of a food processor, combine the chickpeas, freshly squeezed lemon juice, tahini, and minced garlic.

Process the mixture until it forms a thick, grainy paste. Scrape down the sides of the food processor bowl as needed.

With the food processor running, slowly drizzle in the extra virgin olive oil. Continue processing until the mixture becomes smooth and creamy. This may take a few minutes.

Add the ground cumin, paprika, salt, and freshly ground black pepper to the mixture in the food processor.

Process the hummus once more to ensure that the seasonings are well incorporated. Taste and adjust the seasonings if necessary, adding more salt, lemon juice, or olive oil to your liking.

Now, add the chopped fresh herbs to the food processor.

Pulse the food processor a few times to combine the herbs with the hummus. Be careful not to over-process; you want the herbs to be mixed in but still visible.

Scrape Hummus from the food processor bowl into a serving bowl.

Use the back of a spoon to create a well or a swirl in the center of the hummus.

Drizzle a bit more extra virgin olive oil over the top of the hummus, allowing it to pool in the well. Sprinkle paprika over the olive oil for added flavor and a beautiful presentation.

Finally, garnish the hummus with the chopped Kalamata olives. You can also scatter a few additional chopped fresh herbs if you like.

EGGPLANT AND TOMATO BRUSCHETTA

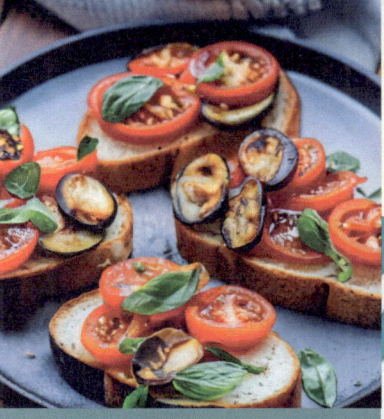

COOKING PROCESS:

Dice the eggplant into small cubes.
Place the diced eggplant in a colander, sprinkle it with salt, and let it sit for about 15-20 minutes. This helps remove excess moisture and bitterness from the eggplant.
After the resting time, rinse the eggplant cubes under cold water and pat them dry with paper towels.
In a large skillet, heat 1/4 cup of extra-virgin olive oil over medium heat.
Add the minced garlic to the skillet and sauté for about 30 seconds until fragrant.
Add the diced eggplant to the skillet and cook, stirring occasionally, until it becomes tender and golden brown, which should take about 10-15 minutes.
Season the eggplant with salt and pepper to taste.
In a mixing bowl, combine the sautéed eggplant, diced tomatoes, chopped fresh basil, and balsamic vinegar.
Drizzle a little extra-virgin olive oil over the mixture for added flavor and moisture.
Toss everything together until the ingredients are well combined.
Preheat your oven's broiler to high.
Place the slices of crusty bread on a baking sheet. Lightly brush each slice with extra-virgin olive oil and rub them with the peeled garlic clove to infuse the bread with garlic flavor.
Place the baking sheet under the broiler for about 1-2 minutes on each side, or until the bread is toasted and golden brown. Keep a close eye on it to prevent burning.
Once the bread is toasted, remove it from the oven.
Spoon the Eggplant and Tomato Bruschetta topping generously onto each slice of toasted bread.
Garnish with fresh basil leaves, if desired.

INGREDIENTS:

FOR THE BRUSCHETTA TOPPING:

- 1 medium eggplant
- 2 medium tomato
- 2 cloves garlic
- 1/4 cup fresh basil leaves
- 1/4 cup extra-virgin olive oil, plus extra for drizzling
- 1 tablespoon balsamic vinegar
- Salt and pepper, to taste

FOR THE BRUSCHETTA BASE:

- 4 large slices of crusty bread (such as baguette or ciabatta)
- 1 clove garlic, peeled Extra-virgin olive oil, for brushing
- Fresh basil leaves, for garnish (optional)

Snacks and Appetizers for Vitality

DATE AND NUT STUFFED BAKED APPLES

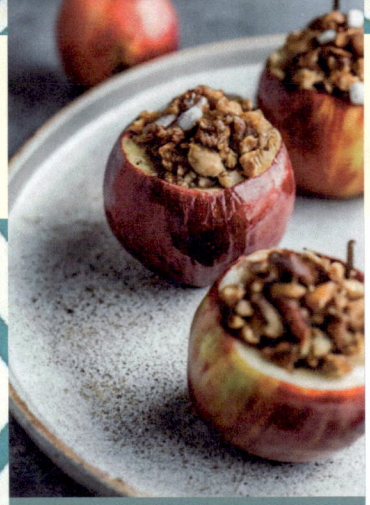

INGREDIENTS:

- 4 large baking apples (such as Granny Smith or Honeycrisp)
- 1/2 cup chopped dates
- 1/2 cup chopped nuts (walnuts or pecans work well)
- 2 tablespoons honey or maple syrup
- 1 teaspoon ground cinnamon
- 1/2 teaspoon vanilla extract (optional)
- A pinch of salt
- 1/2 cup apple juice or water

COOKING PROCESS:

Preheat your oven to 350°F (175°C).
Start by preparing the apples. Wash and dry them thoroughly. Then, use a sharp knife or an apple corer to remove the cores, creating a hollow cavity in each apple. Be careful not to cut through the bottom of the apples; you want to create a well for the stuffing.

In a mixing bowl, combine: 1/2 cup chopped dates, 1/2 cup chopped nuts (walnuts or pecans), 2 tablespoons honey or maple syrup for sweetness, 1 teaspoon ground cinnamon for warm, spiced flavor, 1/2 teaspoon vanilla extract for added aroma and flavor (optional), a pinch of salt for balance.
Mix the ingredients together until they are well combined.

Stuff each cored apple with the date and nut mixture. You can use a spoon to press the mixture into the apples, ensuring they are well filled.

Place the stuffed apples in a baking dish, and pour 1/2 cup of apple juice or water into the bottom of the dish. This helps create a steamy environment and prevents the apples from drying out during baking.

Cover the baking dish with aluminum foil to trap steam and moisture, and then place it in the preheated oven.
Bake the stuffed apples for approximately 35-45 minutes, or until they are tender when pierced with a fork. The baking time may vary depending on the size and type of apples you use.

Once the apples are tender, remove them from the oven and let them cool slightly before serving.

Your Date and Nut Stuffed Baked Apples are now ready to enjoy as a warm and comforting dessert. Serve them as is or with a dollop of Greek yogurt or vanilla ice cream for added richness.

BANANA WALNUT MUFFINS

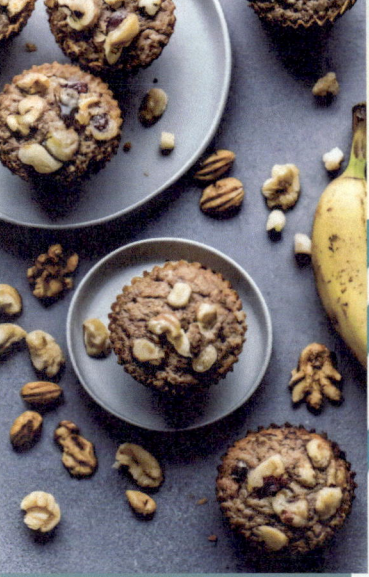

COOKING PROCESS:

Preheat your oven to 350°F (175°C).
Prepare a muffin tin by greasing it with cooking spray or lining it with muffin liners.
In a mixing bowl, peel and mash 2 ripe bananas. You can use a fork or a potato masher for this step.
Add: 1/2 cup granulated sugar, 1 large egg, 1/4 cup melted unsalted butter.
Mix these wet ingredients together until well combined.
In a separate bowl, whisk together the dry ingredients: 1 1/2 cups all-purpose flour, 1 teaspoon baking soda, 1/2 teaspoon baking powder, 1/2 teaspoon salt (if desired), 1/2 teaspoon ground cinnamon (if desired).
Gradually add the dry ingredient mixture to the wet ingredients.
Stir until just combined. Be careful not to overmix; a few lumps are okay.
Gently fold in 1/2 cup chopped walnuts.
The walnuts add a delightful crunch and nutty flavor to the muffins.
Spoon the muffin batter into the prepared muffin tin, filling each cup about two-thirds full.
Optionally, you can sprinkle a few extra chopped walnuts on top of each muffin for added texture and visual appeal.
Bake in the preheated oven for approximately 18-20 minutes or until a toothpick inserted into the center of a muffin comes out clean.
Once baked, remove the muffins from the oven and allow them to cool in the muffin tin for a few minutes.
Transfer the Banana Walnut Muffins to a wire rack to cool completely.
Once cooled, these muffins are ready to enjoy as a tasty breakfast, snack, or dessert.

INGREDIENTS:

- 2 ripe bananas
- 1/2 cup granulated sugar
- 1 large egg
- 1/4 cup unsalted butter
- 1 1/2 cups all-purpose flour
- 1 teaspoon baking soda
- 1/2 teaspoon baking powder
- 1/2 teaspoon salt (optional)
- 1/2 teaspoon ground cinnamon (optional)
- 1/2 cup chopped walnuts (or more to taste)
- Cooking spray or muffin liners

ALMOND AND HONEY RICE PUDDING

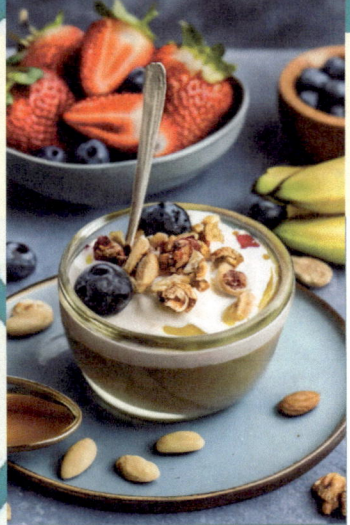

INGREDIENTS:

- 1 cup white rice (long- grain or medium-grain)
- 4 cups milk (whole milk or your preferred milk substitute)
- 1/2 cup granulated sugar (adjust to taste)
- 1/2 teaspoon vanilla extract
- 1/2 cup chopped almonds
- 2 tablespoons honey
- A pinch of salt (optional)
- Ground cinnamon for garnish (optional)

COOKING PROCESS:

Begin by rinsing 1 cup of white rice under cold water until the water runs clear. This removes excess starch and helps prevent the rice from becoming too sticky.

In a large, heavy-bottomed saucepan, combine the rinsed rice and 4 cups of milk. If you prefer a dairy- free option, you can use almond milk, coconut milk, or any milk substitute of your choice.

Add 1/2 cup of granulated sugar to the saucepan. You can adjust the sugar amount to your preferred level of sweetness.

Optionally, add a pinch of salt to enhance the flavors.

Place the saucepan over medium heat and bring the mixture to a simmer while stirring frequently to prevent the rice from sticking to the bottom.

Once the mixture reaches a simmer, reduce the heat to low and cover the saucepan with a lid. Allow the rice to simmer gently for about 20-25 minutes, or until the rice is tender and has absorbed most of the liquid. Stir occasionally to prevent sticking.

When the rice is cooked, remove the saucepan from the heat and stir in 1/2 teaspoon of vanilla extract for added flavor.

In a separate pan, lightly toast 1/2 cup of chopped almonds over low heat until they become fragrant and slightly golden. This will enhance their nutty flavor.

To serve, spoon the warm rice pudding into individual serving bowls.

Drizzle 2 tablespoons of honey over the top of each bowl of rice pudding.

Sprinkle the toasted almonds over the honey-drizzled rice pudding. The almonds add a delightful crunch and nutty flavor.

Optionally, dust the top with a pinch of ground cinnamon for added aroma and flavor.

Your Almond and Honey Rice Pudding is now ready to enjoy as a comforting and indulgent dessert or snack. Serve it warm for the best experience.

LENTIL AND VEGETABLE SOUP

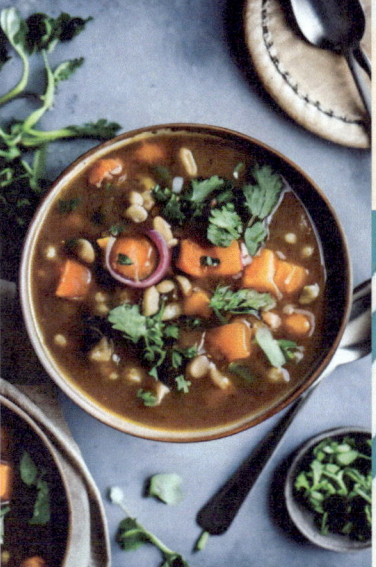

COOKING PROCESS:

Start by rinsing 1 cup of dried green or brown lentils in a fine-mesh strainer under cold running water. Drain and set them aside.
In a large soup pot or Dutch oven, heat a bit of olive oil over medium heat.
Add the chopped onion, diced carrots, and diced celery to the pot.
Sauté the vegetables for about 5 minutes until they begin to soften.
Add the minced garlic to the sautéed vegetables and cook for an additional 30 seconds until fragrant.
Stir in 1 teaspoon of dried thyme and season with salt and pepper to taste.
Add the rinsed and drained lentils to the pot and stir to combine them with the sautéed vegetables.
Pour in the entire can of diced tomatoes, including the juice, and stir again.
Pour in 6 cups of vegetable broth to the pot. Add 1 bay leaf for added flavor.
Stir everything together to ensure all the ingredients are well combined.
Bring the mixture to a boil over high heat.
Once it's boiling, reduce the heat to low, cover the pot, and let the soup simmer for about 25-30 minutes, or until the lentils and vegetables are tender. Stir occasionally.
Taste the soup and adjust the seasoning as needed, adding more salt and pepper if desired.
Remove the bay leaf from the soup before serving.
Ladle the hot Lentil and Vegetable Soup into bowls. Sprinkle each bowl with freshly chopped parsley for a burst of freshness and color.
Enjoy your Lentil and Vegetable Soup as a comforting and nutritious meal, especially on chilly days.

INGREDIENTS:

- 1 cup dried green or brown lentils
- 1 onion
- 2 carrots
- 2 celery stalks
- 2 cloves garlic
- 1 can (15 oz) diced tomatoes
- 6 cups vegetable broth
- 1 teaspoon dried thyme
- 1 bay leaf
- Salt and pepper to taste
- Extra-virgin olive oil
- Fresh parsley (for garnish)

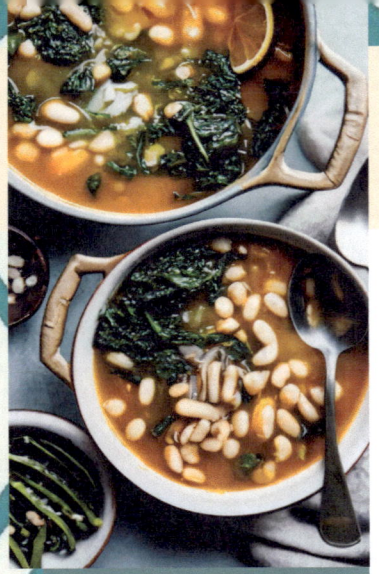

KALE AND WHITE BEAN SOUP

COOKING PROCESS:

Start by washing the kale thoroughly.
Remove the tough stems from the kale leaves and chop the leaves into bite-sized pieces. Set them aside.
In a large soup pot or Dutch oven, heat a bit of olive oil over medium heat.
Add the chopped onion, diced carrots, and diced celery to the pot.
Sauté the vegetables for about 5 minutes until they begin to soften.
Add the minced garlic to the sautéed vegetables and cook for an additional 30 seconds until fragrant.
Stir in 1 teaspoon of dried thyme and season with salt and pepper to taste.
Add the chopped kale to the pot and stir it in with the sautéed vegetables. Pour in the drained and rinsed white beans.
Stir to combine all the ingredients.
Pour in 6 cups of vegetable broth to the pot. Add 1 bay leaf for added flavor. Stir everything together to ensure all the ingredients are well combined. Bring the mixture to a boil over high heat.
Once it's boiling, reduce the heat to low, cover the pot, and let the soup simmer for about 20-25 minutes, or until the kale is tender and the flavors meld together. Stir occasionally.
Taste the soup and adjust the seasoning as needed, adding more salt and pepper if desired.
Remove the bay leaf from the soup before serving.
Ladle the hot Kale and White Bean Soup into bowls.
If desired, sprinkle each bowl with grated Parmesan cheese for extra flavor.
Enjoy your Kale and White Bean Soup as a hearty and nutritious meal, especially on a chilly day.

INGREDIENTS:

- 1 bunch of kale, stems removed and leaves chopped
- 2 cans (15 oz each) white beans (cannellini or Great Northern)
- 1 onion
- 2 carrots
- 2 celery stalks
- 3 cloves garlic
- 6 cups vegetable broth
- 1 bay leaf
- 1 teaspoon dried thyme
- Salt and pepper to taste
- Extra-virgin olive oil
- Grated Parmesan cheese (optional, for garnish)

BARLEY AND MUSHROOM SOUP

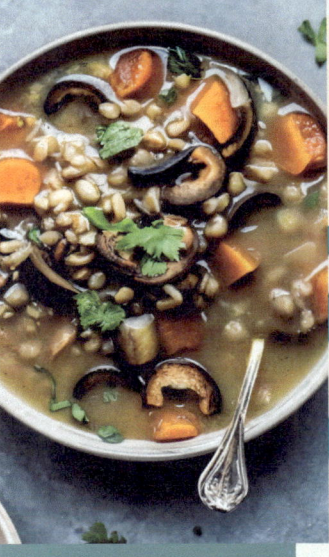

COOKING PROCESS:

Start by rinsing 1 cup of pearl barley under cold running water in a fine-mesh strainer. Drain and set it aside.
In a large soup pot or Dutch oven, heat a bit of olive oil over medium heat.
Add the chopped onion, diced carrots, and diced celery to the pot.
Sauté the vegetables for about 5 minutes until they begin to soften.
Add the minced garlic to the sautéed vegetables and cook for an additional 30 seconds until fragrant.
Stir in 1 teaspoon of dried thyme and season with salt and pepper to taste.
Add the sliced mushrooms to the pot.
Continue sautéing for about 5-7 minutes until the mushrooms release their moisture and start to brown. Stir occasionally.
Combine Barley and Vegetables:
Add the rinsed pearl barley to the pot and stir it in with the sautéed vegetables and mushrooms.
Pour in 6 cups of vegetable broth to the pot.
Add 2 bay leaves for added flavor.
Stir everything together to ensure all the ingredients are well combined.
Bring the mixture to a boil over high heat.
Once it's boiling, reduce the heat to low, cover the pot, and let the soup simmer for about 30-35 minutes, or until the barley is tender and the flavors meld together. Stir occasionally.
Taste the soup and adjust the seasoning as needed, adding more salt and pepper if desired.
Remove the bay leaves from the soup before serving.
Ladle the hot Barley and Mushroom Soup into bowls. Sprinkle each bowl with freshly chopped parsley for a burst of freshness and color.
Enjoy your Barley and Mushroom Soup as a hearty and wholesome meal, perfect for a chilly day.

INGREDIENTS:

- 1 cup pearl barley
- 8 oz mushrooms
- 1 onion
- 2 carrots
- 2 celery stalks
- 3 cloves garlic
- 6 cups vegetable broth
- 2 bay leaves
- 1 teaspoon dried thyme
- Salt and pepper to taste
- Extra-virgin olive oil
- Fresh parsley (for garnish)

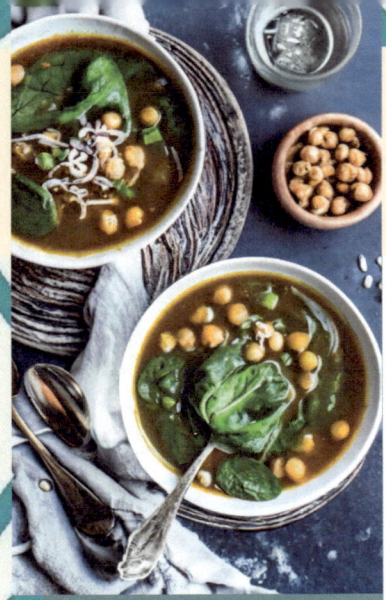

SPINACH AND CHICKPEA SOUP

INGREDIENTS:

- 1 can (15 oz) chickpeas
- 1 onio
- 2 cloves garlic
- 2 carrots
- 2 celery stalks
- 6 cups vegetable broth
- 8 oz fresh spinach leaves
- 1 teaspoon dried thyme
- Salt and pepper to taste
- Extra-virgin olive oil

COOKING PROCESS:

Start bIn a large soup pot or Dutch oven, heat a bit of olive oil over medium heat.
Add the chopped onion, diced carrots, and diced celery to the pot.
Sauté the vegetables for about 5 minutes until they begin to soften.
Add the minced garlic to the sautéed vegetables and cook for an additional 30 seconds until fragrant.
Stir in 1 teaspoon of dried thyme and season with salt and pepper to taste.
Add the drained and rinsed chickpeas to the pot. Pour in 6 cups of vegetable broth.
Bring the mixture to a boil over high heat.
Once it's boiling, reduce the heat to low, cover the pot, and let the soup simmer for about 15-20 minutes to melt the flavors.
If you prefer a smoother texture, you can use an immersion blender to partially blend the soup while it's still in the pot.
Alternatively, transfer a portion of the soup to a blender, blend until smooth, and then return it to the pot.
Be cautious when blending hot soup.
Stir in the chopped fresh spinach leaves.
Allow the spinach to wilt and cook in the hot soup for about 2-3 minutes.
Taste the soup and adjust the seasoning as needed, adding more salt and pepper if desired.
Ladle the hot Spinach and Chickpea Soup into bowls.
If desired, sprinkle each bowl with grated Parmesan cheese for added flavor.
Enjoy your Spinach and Chickpea Soup as a nutritious and comforting meal, perfect for a satisfying lunch or dinner.

CABBAGE AND POTATO SOUP

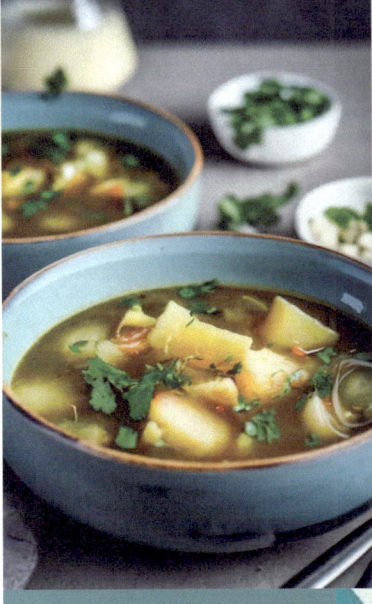

COOKING PROCESS:

Start by shredding a small head of cabbage. Remove the tough outer leaves, cut it into quarters, and then thinly slice it.
Set the shredded cabbage aside.
In a large soup pot or Dutch oven, heat a bit of olive oil over medium heat.
Add the chopped onion and diced potatoes to the pot.
Sauté for about 5 minutes until the onions are translucent and the potatoes start to soften.
Add the minced garlic to the sautéed vegetables and cook for an additional 30 seconds until fragrant.
Stir in 1 teaspoon of dried thyme and season with salt and pepper to taste.
Add the shredded cabbage to the pot and stir it in with the sautéed vegetables and potatoes.
Pour in 6 cups of vegetable broth to the pot.
Add 2 bay leaves for added flavor.
Stir everything together to ensure all the ingredients are well combined.
Bring the mixture to a boil over high heat.
Once it's boiling, reduce the heat to low, cover the pot, and let the soup simmer for about 25-30 minutes, or until the potatoes are tender, and the flavors meld together.
Stir occasionally.
Taste the soup and adjust the seasoning as needed, adding more salt and pepper if desired.
Remove the bay leaves from the soup before serving.
Ladle the hot Cabbage and Potato Soup into bowls.
Sprinkle each bowl with freshly chopped dill for added flavor and a touch of freshness.
Enjoy your Cabbage and Potato Soup as a hearty and wholesome meal, perfect for a chilly day.

INGREDIENTS:

- 1 small head of cabbage
- 4 potatoes
- 1 onion
- 2 cloves garlic
- 6 cups vegetable broth
- 2 bay leaves
- 1 teaspoon dried thyme
- Salt and pepper to taste
- Extra-virgin olive oil
- Fresh dill (for garnish)

TOMATO LENTIL SOUP

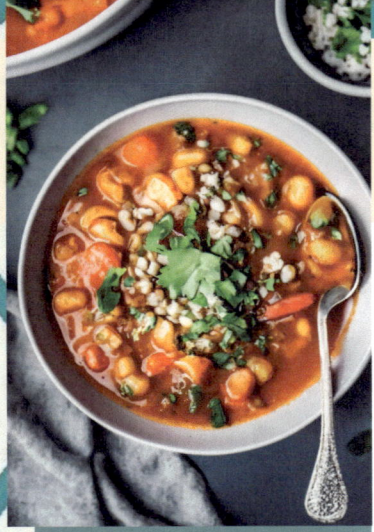

INGREDIENTS:

- 1 cup dried brown or green lentils
- 1 onion
- 2 cloves garlic
- 2 carrots
- 2 celery stalks
- 1 can (15 oz) diced tomatoes
- 6 cups vegetable broth
- 1 teaspoon dried oregano
- 1 teaspoon dried basil
- Salt and pepper to taste
- Extra-virgin olive oil
- Fresh basil leaves (for garnish)

COOKING PROCESS:

Start by rinsing 1 cup of dried brown or green lentils under cold running water in a fine-mesh strainer. Drain and set them aside.

In a large soup pot or Dutch oven, heat a bit of olive oil over medium heat.

Add the chopped onion, diced carrots, and diced celery to the pot.

Sauté the vegetables for about 5 minutes until they begin to soften.

Add the minced garlic to the sautéed vegetables and cook for an additional 30 seconds until fragrant.

Stir in 1 teaspoon of dried oregano and 1 teaspoon of dried basil. Season with salt and pepper to taste.

Add the rinsed and drained lentils to the pot.

Pour in the entire can of diced tomatoes, including the juice.

Stir everything together to combine the ingredients.

Pour in 6 cups of vegetable broth to the pot.

Stir to ensure all the ingredients are well mixed. Bring the mixture to a boil over high heat.

Once it's boiling, reduce the heat to low, cover the pot, and let the soup simmer for about 25-30 minutes, or until the lentils are tender and the flavors meld together.

Stir occasionally.

Taste the soup and adjust the seasoning as needed, adding more salt and pepper if desired.

Ladle the hot Tomato Lentil Soup into bowls. Sprinkle each bowl with freshly chopped basil leaves for added flavor and a touch of freshness.

Enjoy your Tomato Lentil Soup as a nutritious and comforting meal, perfect for a satisfying lunch or dinner.

SWEET POTATO AND GINGER SOUP

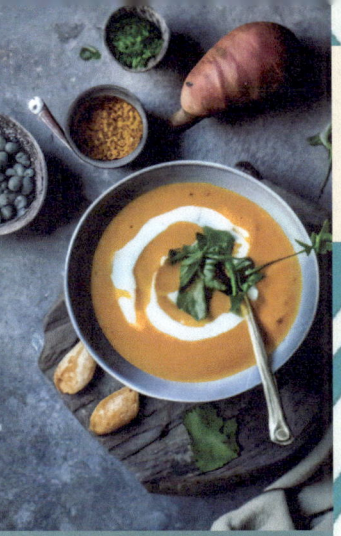

COOKING PROCESS:

Start by peeling and dicing 3 large sweet potatoes into small, even-sized pieces. Set them aside.
In a large soup pot or Dutch oven, heat a bit of olive oil over medium heat.
Add the chopped onion and diced sweet potatoes to the pot.
Sauté for about 5 minutes until the onions are translucent and the sweet potatoes start to soften.
Add the minced garlic and minced fresh ginger to the sautéed vegetables.
Cook for an additional 1-2 minutes until fragrant, stirring constantly.
Sprinkle 1 teaspoon of ground cinnamon and 1/2 teaspoon of ground nutmeg over the sautéed vegetables.
Season with salt and pepper to taste.
Pour in 6 cups of vegetable broth to the pot.
Stir to ensure all the ingredients are well mixed.
Bring the mixture to a boil over high heat.
Once it's boiling, reduce the heat to low, cover the pot, and let the soup simmer for about 20- 25 minutes, or until the sweet potatoes are tender and the flavors meld together.
Stir occasionally.
Taste the soup and adjust the seasoning as needed, adding more salt, pepper, or spices if desired.
Use an immersion blender to puree the soup until smooth.
Alternatively, transfer the soup in batches to a blender, blend until smooth, and then return it to the pot. Be cautious when blending hot soup.
Ladle the hot Sweet Potato and Ginger Soup into bowls.
Garnish each bowl with fresh cilantro leaves for added flavor and a touch of freshness.
Enjoy your Sweet Potato and Ginger Soup as a comforting and flavorful meal, perfect for a cozy dinner.

INGREDIENTS:

- 3 large sweet potatoes
- 1 onion
- 2 cloves garlic
- 1-inch piece of fresh ginger
- 6 cups vegetable broth
- 1 teaspoon ground cinnamon
- 1/2 teaspoon ground nutmeg
- Salt and pepper to taste
- Extra-virgin olive oil
- Fresh cilantro leaves (for garnish)

QUINOA AND VEGETABLE SOUP

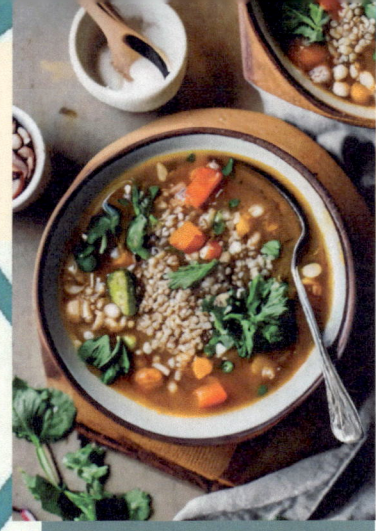

INGREDIENTS:

- 1 cup quinoa
- 2 carrots
- 2 celery stalks
- 1 onion
- 2 cloves garlic
- 6 cups vegetable broth
- 1 can (15 oz) diced tomatoes
- 1 teaspoon dried thyme
- 1 bay leaf
- Salt and pepper to taste
- Extra-virgin olive oil
- Fresh parsley (for garnish)

COOKING PROCESS:

Start by rinsing 1 cup of quinoa in a fine-mesh strainer under cold running water. Drain and set it aside.

In a large soup pot or Dutch oven, heat a bit of olive oil over medium heat.

Add the chopped onion, diced carrots, and diced celery to the pot.

Sauté the vegetables for about 5 minutes until they begin to soften.

Add the minced garlic to the sautéed vegetables and cook for an additional 30 seconds until fragrant.

Stir in 1 teaspoon of dried thyme and season with salt and pepper to taste.

Add the rinsed and drained quinoa to the pot and stir it in with the sautéed vegetables.

Pour in 6 cups of vegetable broth to the pot.

Add 1 bay leaf for added flavor.

Stir everything together to ensure all the ingredients are well combined.

Pour in the entire can of diced tomatoes, including the juice.

Stir to incorporate the tomatoes into the soup.

Bring the mixture to a boil over high heat.

Once it's boiling, reduce the heat to low, cover the pot, and let the soup simmer for about 15-20 minutes, or until the quinoa is cooked and the flavors meld together.

Stir occasionally.

Taste the soup and adjust the seasoning as needed, adding more salt and pepper if desired.

Remove the bay leaf from the soup before serving.

Ladle the hot Quinoa and Vegetable Soup into bowls.

Sprinkle each bowl with freshly chopped parsley for added freshness and color.

Enjoy your Quinoa and Vegetable Soup as a nutritious and satisfying meal, perfect for lunch or dinner.

TURMERIC AND CAULIFLOWER SOUP

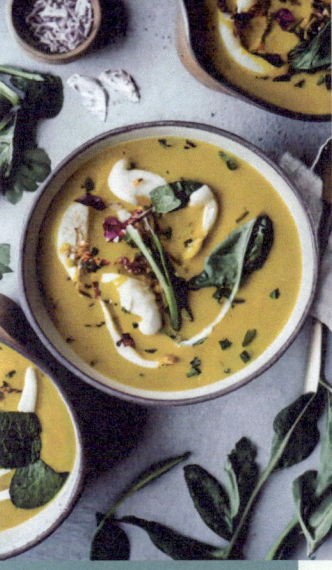

COOKING PROCESS:

Start by cutting 1 head of cauliflower into florets. You can break it into small, bite-sized pieces. Set them aside.
In a large soup pot or Dutch oven, heat a bit of olive oil over medium heat.
Add the chopped onion and cauliflower florets to the pot. Sauté for about 5 minutes until the onions are translucent and the cauliflower starts to turn golden brown.
Add the minced garlic and minced fresh turmeric (or ground turmeric) to the sautéed vegetables. Cook for an additional 1-2 minutes until fragrant, stirring constantly.
Sprinkle 1 teaspoon of ground cumin over the sautéed vegetables. Season with salt and pepper to taste.
Pour in 6 cups of vegetable broth to the pot.
Stir to ensure all the ingredients are well mixed. Bring the mixture to a boil over high heat.
Once it's boiling, reduce the heat to low, cover the pot, and let the soup simmer for about 20-25 minutes, or until the cauliflower is tender and the flavors meld together. Stir occasionally.
Use an immersion blender to puree the soup until smooth. Alternatively, transfer the soup in batches to a blender, blend until smooth, and then return it to the pot.
Be cautious when blending hot soup.
Pour in the entire can of coconut milk and stir to combine it with the soup. This adds creaminess and a subtle coconut flavor.
Taste the soup and adjust the seasoning as needed, adding more salt and pepper if desired.
Ladle the hot Turmeric and Cauliflower Soup into bowls.
Garnish each bowl with fresh cilantro leaves for added flavor and a vibrant touch.
Enjoy your Turmeric and Cauliflower Soup as a comforting and flavorful meal, perfect for a cozy dinner.

INGREDIENTS:

- 1 head of cauliflower
- 1 onion
- 2 cloves garlic
- 1-inch piece of fresh turmeric, peeled and minced (or 1 teaspoon ground turmeric)
- 6 cups vegetable broth
- 1 can (15 oz) coconut milk
- 1 teaspoon ground cumin
- Salt and pepper to taste
- Extra-virgin olive oil
- Fresh cilantro leaves (for garnish)

GREEN PEA AND MINT SOUP

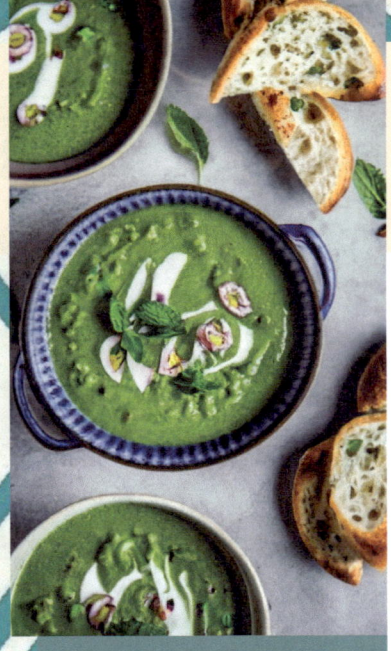

INGREDIENTS:

- 4 cups frozen green peas
- 1 onion
- 2 cloves garlic
- 6 cups vegetable broth
- 1/2 cup fresh mint leaves, plus extra for garnish
- 1/2 cup plain Greek yogurt (or dairy-free alternative)
- Salt and pepper to taste
- Extra-virgin olive oil

COOKING PROCESS:

In a large soup pot or Dutch oven, heat a bit of olive oil over medium heat.
Add the chopped onion to the pot and sauté for about 5 minutes until it becomes translucent.
Add the minced garlic to the sautéed onions and cook for an additional 30 seconds until fragrant.
Add the frozen green peas to the pot and stir to combine with the sautéed onions and garlic.
Pour in 6 cups of vegetable broth to the pot.
Stir everything together to ensure the peas are submerged in the broth.
Bring the mixture to a boil over high heat.
Once it's boiling, reduce the heat to low, cover the pot, and let the soup simmer for about 10-15 minutes, or until the peas are tender and heated through.
Stir in 1/2 cup of fresh mint leaves.
These will add a fresh and bright flavor to the soup.
Use an immersion blender to puree the soup until smooth. Alternatively, transfer the soup in batches to a blender, blend until smooth, and then return it to the pot.
Be cautious when blending hot soup.
Stir in 1/2 cup of plain Greek yogurt (or a dairy-free alternative) to the soup.
This will add creaminess and a touch of tang.
Taste the soup and adjust the seasoning as needed, adding more salt and pepper if desired.
Ladle the hot Green Pea and Mint Soup into bowls.
Garnish each bowl with a sprig of fresh mint leaves for added freshness and presentation.
Enjoy your Green Pea and Mint Soup as a refreshing and flavorful meal, perfect for a light lunch or dinner.

VEGAN MISO SOUP

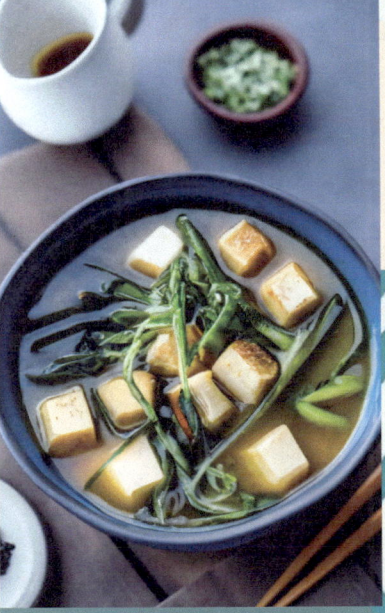

COOKING PROCESS:

Start by preparing the dried seaweed (wakame).
Place 2 tablespoons of dried seaweed in a small bowl of cold water and let it soak for about 5 minutes or until it rehydrates and becomes tender.
Drain the seaweed and set it aside.
In a medium-sized pot, bring 4 cups of water to a gentle simmer.
Do not bring it to a rolling boil.
Add the rehydrated seaweed to the simmering water and continue to cook for about 2-3 minutes until the seaweed is fully rehydrated and tender.
Add 1/2 cup of cubed tofu to the soup.
Let it simmer for an additional 2-3 minutes until the tofu is heated through.
In a small bowl, dissolve 4 tablespoons of miso paste in a few tablespoons of hot water to create a smooth miso mixture.
This helps prevent lumps in the soup.
Gradually add the miso mixture to the pot while stirring gently.
Avoid boiling the miso soup once the miso paste has been added, as boiling can reduce its flavor.
If desired, you can add 1 tablespoon of soy sauce to enhance the umami flavor of the soup.
Stir to combine.
Garnish each bowl with thinly sliced green onions and a pinch of bonito flakes, if desired.
The bonito flakes add a subtle smoky flavor.
Serve the miso soup hot and enjoy it as a comforting and flavorful appetizer or part of a larger Japanese meal.

INGREDIENTS:

- 4 cups water
- 4 tablespoons miso paste (white or red, according to preference)
- 2 tablespoons dried seaweed (wakame)
- 1/2 cup tofu
- 2 green onions, thinly sliced
- 1 tablespoon soy sauce (optional, for extra flavor)
- A pinch of bonito flakes (katsuobushi) for garnish (optional)

MISO SOUP WITH TOFU AND SEAWEED

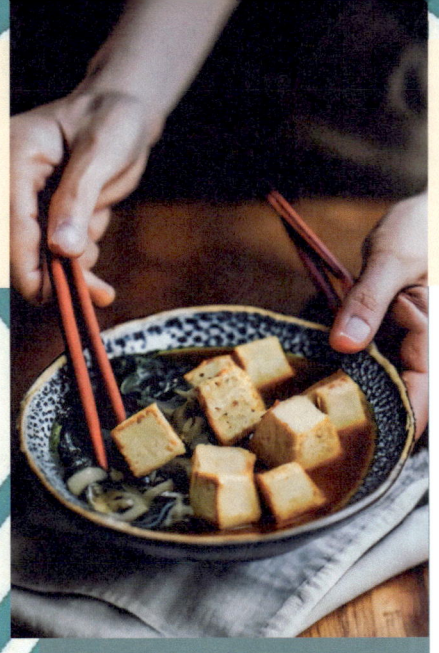

INGREDIENTS:

- 4 cups dashi stock (you can use instant dashi granules or make your own with kombu seaweed and bonito flakes)
- 1/2 cup miso paste (white or red, depending on your preference)
- 1/2 cup cubed tofu (silken or firm)
- 2-3 tablespoons dried wakame seaweed (rehydrated in water)
- 2-3 green onions
- 1-2 shiitake mushrooms (for added flavor, optional)
- 1 teaspoon mirin (Japanese sweet rice wine, optional)
- 1 teaspoon soy sauce (for extra flavor, optional)

COOKING PROCESS:

If you're using instant dashi granules, follow the package instructions to make 4 cups of dashi stock.

If you're making your own dashi, simmer a piece of kombu seaweed (about 2 inches square) in 4 cups of water for about 10-15 minutes. Remove the kombu and add 1/4 cup of bonito flakes.

Simmer for an additional 5 minutes, then strain the stock.

Place the dried wakame seaweed in a small bowl and cover it with warm water.

Let it sit for about 5 minutes until it rehydrates.

Drain and set aside.

Cut the tofu into small cubes and set aside.

If you're using shiitake mushrooms, thinly slice them and set them aside.

In a large saucepan, heat the dashi stock over medium heat. If you're using mirin and soy sauce for extra flavor, add them to the stock now.

In a small bowl, dissolve the miso paste in a ladleful of hot dashi stock. Stir until the miso is fully dissolved.

Once the dashi stock is hot (but not boiling), add the tofu cubes and sliced shiitake mushrooms (if using). Simmer for about 2-3 minutes.

Add the rehydrated wakame seaweed to the soup and simmer for an additional 1-2 minutes.

Turn off the heat, and then stir in the dissolved miso paste. Be careful not to boil the soup once the miso is added, as high heat can reduce the miso's flavor.

Ladle the miso soup into bowls. Garnish with thinly sliced green onions.

Serve hot as a comforting and nutritious soup.

MINESTRONE SOUP

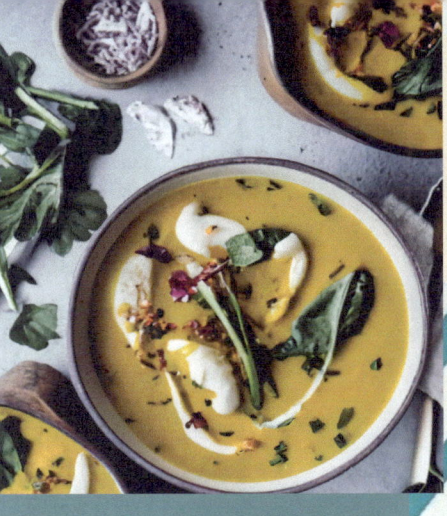

COOKING PROCESS:

In a large pot or Dutch oven, heat the olive oil over medium heat.
Add the chopped onion and garlic, and sauté for about 2 minutes or until they become fragrant and translucent.
Add the diced carrots, diced celery, diced zucchini, and cut green beans to the pot. Sauté for an additional 5 minutes, stirring occasionally until the vegetables start to soften.
Pour in the diced tomatoes, kidney beans, and cannellini beans (make sure to drain and rinse them beforehand).
Stir to combine.
Pour in the vegetable or chicken broth. Add the dried basil, dried oregano, dried thyme, salt, and black pepper to taste.
Stir well to incorporate all the ingredients.
Increase the heat to high and bring the soup to a boil.
Once the soup is boiling, add the small pasta of your choice.
Reduce the heat to medium-low and let the soup simmer for about 10-12 minutes or until the pasta is cooked al dente and the vegetables are tender.
Stir in the chopped fresh spinach or kale and simmer for an additional 2-3 minutes until the greens are wilted.
Taste the soup and adjust the seasoning with more salt and pepper if needed.
Ladle the hot Italian Minestrone Soup into bowls.
If desired, garnish with grated Parmesan cheese and fresh basil leaves.
Serve the soup hot and enjoy the comforting flavors of this Italian classic.

INGREDIENTS:

- 2 tablespoons olive oil
- 1 medium onion
- 2 cloves garlic
- 2 carrots
- 2 celery stalks
- 1 zucchini
- 1 cup green beans, cut into 1-inch pieces
- 1 can (15 ounces) diced tomatoes
- 1 can (15 ounces) kidney beans, drained and rinsed
- 1 can (15 ounces) cannellini beans
- 8 cups vegetable or chicken broth
- 1 cup small pasta (such as ditalini or elbow macaroni)
- 1 teaspoon dried basil
- 1 teaspoon dried oregano
- 1/2 teaspoon dried thyme
- Salt and black pepper to taste
- 2 cups chopped fresh spinach or kale
- Grated Parmesan cheese for serving (optional)
- Fresh basil leaves for garnish (optional)

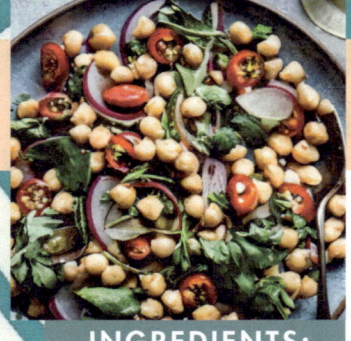

MEDITERRANEAN CHICKPEA SALAD

INGREDIENTS:

- 2 cans (15 oz each) chickpeas
- 1 cucumber
- 2 tomatoes
- 1 red onion
- 1/2 cup Kalamata olives pitted
- 1/2 cup feta cheese
- Fresh parsley and mint
- Juice of 2 lemons
- 3 tbsp extra-virgin olive oil
- Salt and pepper

COOKING PROCESS:

Start by draining and rinsing cans of chickpeas under cold running water in a fine-mesh strainer. Allow them to drain thoroughly.

Dice cucumber and tomatoes into small, bite-sized pieces. Finely chop the red onion, slice Kalamata olives, and crumble feta cheese. Gather fresh parsley and mint leaves and chop them coarsely. You can use as much or as little as you prefer, depending on your taste.

In a small bowl, whisk together the juice of lemons and extra-virgin olive oil. This will be your salad dressing.

In a large mixing bowl, combine the drained chickpeas, cucumber, tomatoes, onion, olives, and crumbled feta cheese. Add the parsley and mint to the bowl.

Drizzle the prepared lemon and olive oil dressing over the salad mixture. Season the salad with salt and pepper to taste. Gently toss all the ingredients together until they are well coated with the dressing.

Cover the bowl with plastic wrap or a lid and refrigerate the salad for at least 30 minutes before serving. Chilling allows the flavors to meld.

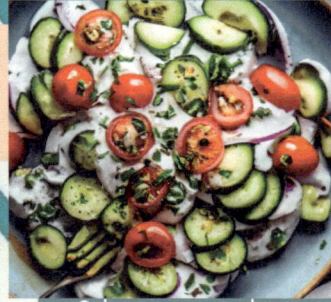

- 2 large cucumbers
- 1 cup Greek yogurt
- 2 cloves garlic
- 1 tablespoon extra-virgin olive oil
- 1 tbsp juice of lemon
- 2 tbsp fresh dill
- Salt and pepper
- 1/2 cup crumbled feta cheese (optional)
- 1/4 cup Kalamata olives pitted (optional)
- Cherry tomatoes for garnish (optional)

TZATZIKI CUCUMBER SALAD

Start by preparing the cucumbers. Wash and peel the cucumbers if desired. Thinly slice them into rounds or half-moons. You should have approximately 4 cups of sliced cucumbers.

In a mixing bowl, combine 1 1/2 cups of Greek yogurt, minced garlic, chopped fresh dill, and lemon juice. Mix these ingredients together thoroughly to create a creamy dressing for the salad.

Add the sliced cucumbers to the yogurt dressing. Gently toss them until the cucumber slices are evenly coated with the dressing. This step creates the base of the salad.

Stir in the fresh dill and season the salad with salt and pepper to taste. If desired, gently fold in the crumbled feta cheese and sliced Kalamata olives for extra flavor.

Chill the salad in the refrigerator for at least 30 minutes before serving to allow the flavors to meld.

Garnish with cherry tomatoes before serving, if you like. This salad is perfect as a side dish with grilled meats, pita bread, or as a refreshing accompaniment to Mediterranean-inspired meals.

OKINAWAN SEARED AHI TUNA SALAD

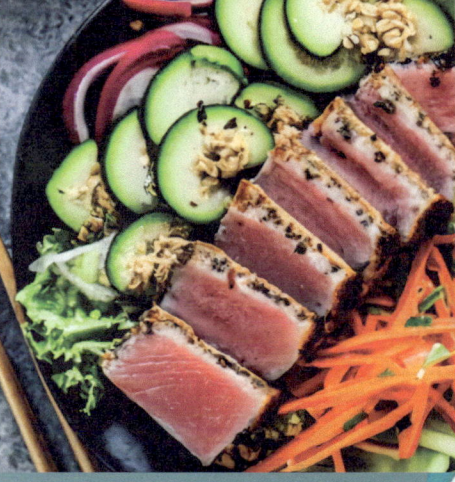

COOKING PROCESS:

In a bowl, combine soy sauce, sesame oil, minced garlic, grated ginger, sesame seeds, salt, and black pepper.
This will be your marinade.
Place the tuna steaks in a shallow dish and pour the marinade over them.
Make sure the tuna is well coated.
Cover and refrigerate for at least 30 minutes to marinate.
Heat a grill or a skillet over high heat. Make sure it's very hot.
Remove the tuna steaks from the marinade and let any excess drip off.
Sear the tuna steaks for about 1-2 minutes per side for rare, or longer if you prefer it more well-done.
The tuna should have a seared crust while the center remains pink.
Once done, remove the tuna from the heat and let it rest for a minute. Then, slice the tuna into thin strips.
Preparing a Salad. Thinly slice cucumber, bell pepper, red onion. Peel and julienne the carrot.
Dice the avocado. In a large salad bowl, combine the mixed greens, cucumber, carrot, red bell pepper, red onion, and avocado.
In a separate bowl, whisk together the soy sauce, rice vinegar, honey, grated ginger, sesame oil, lime juice, salt, and black pepper.
This is your dressing.
Pour the dressing over the salad and toss to combine.
Arrange the dressed salad on serving plates.
Top with the sliced seared ahi tuna.
Garnish with fresh cilantro.
Serve immediately and enjoy your Okinawan Seared Ahi Tuna Salad!

INGREDIENTS:

For the Tuna:
- 4 Ahi tuna steaks (about 6-8 ounces each)
- 2 tablespoons soy sauce
- 2 tablespoons sesame oil
- 2 cloves garlic
- 1 teaspoon fresh ginger
- 1 tablespoon sesame seeds
- Salt and black pepper to taste

For the Salad:
- 8 cups mixed salad greens (such as lettuce, arugula, and spinach)
- 1 cucumber
- 1 carrot
- 1 red bell pepper
- 1/2 red onion
- 1 avocado
- 1/4 cup fresh cilantro (for garnish)

For the Dressing:
- 1/4 cup soy sauce
- 2 tablespoons rice vinegar
- 1 tablespoon honey
- 1 teaspoon fresh ginger
- 2 tablespoons sesame oil
- 1 tablespoon lime juice
- Salt and black pepper to taste)

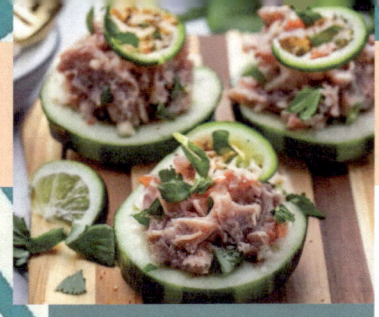

CUCUMBER CUPS WITH TUNA SALAD

INGREDIENTS:

Tuna Salad:
- 2 cans (5 ounces each) of canned tuna
- 1/4 cup mayonnaise (you can use light or Greek yogurt as a healthier alternative)
- 1 celery stalk
- 1/4 red onion
- 2 tablespoons fresh dill Juice of 1 lemon
- Salt and pepper, to taste

For the Cucumber Cups:
- 2 large cucumbers
- Fresh parsley or dill leaves (for garnish)

COOKING PROCESS:

Drain the liquid from the canned tuna.
In a mixing bowl, combine the drained canned tuna, mayonnaise (or yogurt), finely chopped celery, finely chopped red onion, chopped fresh dill, and the juice of lemon.
Season the tuna salad with salt and pepper to taste. Start with a pinch of each and adjust based on your preference. Mix all these ingredients thoroughly to create the tuna salad.
Wash and dry the cucumbers. Trim off both ends of each cucumber. Cut each cucumber into equal-sized segments, about 2 inches long.
Using a small spoon or a melon baller, scoop out the seeds and create a small well in each cucumber segment, creating a "cucumber cup."
Fill each cucumber cup with a spoonful of the prepared tuna salad. Fill them generously but not to the point of overflowing.
Garnish the Cucumber Cups with Tuna Salad by placing a fresh parsley or dill leaf on top of each cup. Arrange the Cucumber Cups with Tuna Salad on a serving platter or individual plates.

CAPRESE SALAD

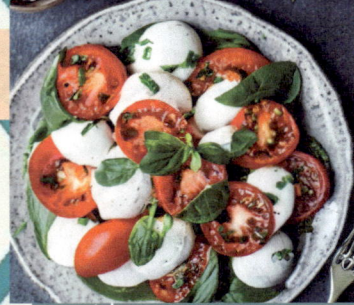

- 4 large ripe tomatoes
- 1 ball fresh mozzarella cheese
- 12-16 fresh basil leaves
- 4 tablespoons extra-virgin olive oil
- 2 tablespoons balsamic vinegar
- Salt and freshly ground black pepper, to taste

Begin by slicing 4 large ripe tomatoes and 1 ball of fresh mozzarella cheese into approximately 1/4-inch thick rounds. You should have enough slices for 4 portions.
On a large serving platter or individual salad plates, arrange the tomato and mozzarella slices alternately, creating a visually appealing pattern.
Tuck fresh basil leaves between the tomato and mozzarella slices. Basil not only adds a burst of flavor but also enhances the visual appeal of the salad. You can use 12-16 fresh basil leaves for 4 servings.
In a small bowl, whisk together 4 tablespoons of extra-virgin olive oil and 2 tablespoons of balsamic vinegar until well combined. This dressing will provide a rich and tangy contrast to the salad.
Drizzle the olive oil and balsamic vinegar dressing generously over the tomato and mozzarella slices. Ensure that each portion receives an even coating of the dressing. Season with salt and pepper.

Mediterranean Tabbouleh Salad

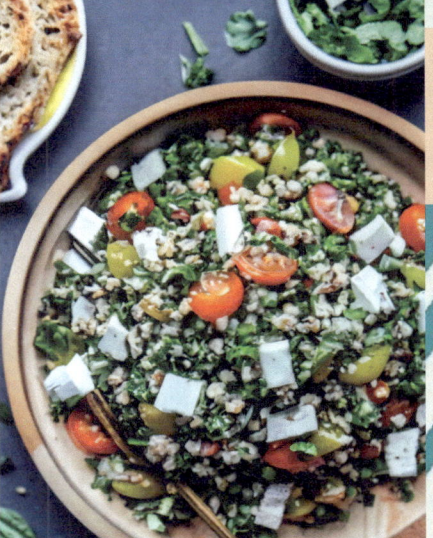

COOKING PROCESS:

Place the bulgur wheat in a heatproof bowl. Pour 1 1/2 cups of boiling water over the bulgur.
Cover the bowl with a lid or plastic wrap and let it sit for about 20-30 minutes, or until the bulgur is tender and has absorbed all the water.
Fluff the cooked bulgur with a fork and let it cool to room temperature.
While the bulgur is cooling, prepare the fresh ingredients.
Finely chop the fresh parsley and mint leaves.
Dice the tomatoes, cucumber, green onions, and red onion (if using).
Chop the Kalamata olives.
If you're including feta cheese, crumble it and set it aside.
In a large mixing bowl, combine the cooled bulgur with the chopped parsley, mint, tomatoes, cucumber, green onions, red onion (if using), and Kalamata olives.
Gently toss the ingredients to mix them evenly.
In a small bowl, whisk together the extra-virgin olive oil, fresh lemon juice, minced garlic (if using), salt, and pepper.
Taste the dressing and adjust the seasoning as needed.
You can add more lemon juice, salt, or pepper to suit your taste.
Drizzle the prepared dressing over the salad mixture.
Gently toss the salad to coat all the ingredients with the dressing. Make sure everything is well combined.
If you're including feta cheese, sprinkle it over the top of the salad and gently mix it in.
Cover the bowl with plastic wrap and refrigerate the Mediterranean Tabbouleh Salad for at least 30 minutes before serving.
This salad is best served chilled.

INGREDIENTS:

For the Salad:

- 1 cup bulgur wheat
- 1 1/2 cups boiling water
- 2 cups fresh parsley
- 1 cup fresh mint leaves
- 2 ripe tomatoes
- 1 cucumber
- 4 green onions (scallions)
- 1/4 cup red onion chopped (optional)
- 1/4 cup Kalamata olives pitted
- 1/4 cup crumbled feta cheese (optional)
- Salt and pepper, to taste

For the Dressing:

- 1/4 cup extra-virgin olive oil
- 1/4 cup fresh lemon juice (about 2 lemons)
- 1 clove garlic (optional)
- Salt and pepper, to taste

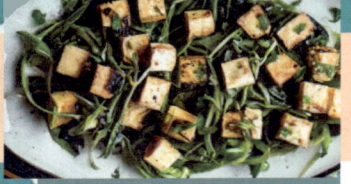

OKINAWAN TOFU AND SEAWEED SALAD

INGREDIENTS:

For the Salad:
- 1 block (14 ounces) firm tofu drained
- 1 cup dried wakame seaweed
- 1 cucumber
- 1/2 red onion
- 2 green onions
- 1 tbsp sesame seeds, toasted (optional)
- 1/4 cup fresh cilantro leaves

For the Dressing:
- 3 tbsp soy sauce
- 2 tbsp rice vinegar
- 1 tbsp sesame oil
- 1 tbsp honey or agave nectar
- 1 clove garlic
- 1 tsp fresh ginger

COOKING PROCESS:

Place the dried wakame seaweed in a bowl of warm water and let it soak for about 5 minutes or until it's rehydrated.

Drain and squeeze out excess water. Set aside.

Cut the firm tofu into small cubes and set them aside.

In a small bowl, whisk together the soy sauce, rice vinegar, sesame oil, honey (or agave nectar), minced garlic, minced ginger, and toasted sesame seeds (if using). Set the dressing aside.

In a large mixing bowl, combine the rehydrated wakame seaweed, sliced cucumber, thinly sliced red onion, and thinly sliced green onions.

Gently add the cubed tofu to the vegetable mixture.

Pour the prepared dressing over the salad ingredients.

Carefully toss all the ingredients until the salad is well coated with the dressing. Refrigerate the salad for about 30 minutes to allow the flavors to meld.

Just before serving, sprinkle toasted sesame seeds (if using) and fresh cilantro leaves over the salad for added flavor and presentation.

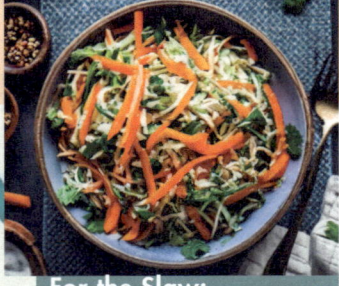

CABBAGE AND CARROT SLAW

For the Slaw:
- 1/2 head of green cabbage
- 2 large carrots
- 1/4 cup red onion
- 1/4 cup fresh parsley
- 1/4 cup roasted sunflower seeds

For the Dressing
- 1/4 cup mayonnaise (or Greek yogurt)
- 2 tbsp apple cider vinegar
- 1 tbsp honey
- 1 tsp Dijon mustard
- Salt and pepper

Thinly shred the green cabbage. You can use a sharp knife or a mandoline slicer for this. Grate or julienne the carrots. Finely chop the red onion. If you're including fresh parsley and roasted sunflower seeds, chop the parsley and set aside the sunflower seeds for garnish.

In a small bowl, whisk together the mayonnaise (or Greek yogurt), apple cider vinegar, honey, Dijon mustard, salt, and pepper. Taste the dressing and adjust the sweetness, acidity, or seasoning to your liking. You can add more honey or vinegar if needed.

In a large mixing bowl, combine the shredded cabbage, grated or julienned carrots, and finely chopped red onion.

Pour the prepared dressing over the vegetables in the mixing bowl. Toss the slaw thoroughly to ensure that the dressing coats all the ingredients evenly.

Cover the bowl with plastic wrap and refrigerate the Cabbage and Carrot Slaw for at least 30 minutes before serving. Chilling allows the flavors to meld and makes the slaw more refreshing.

Just before serving, garnish the slaw with chopped fresh parsley and roasted sunflower seeds, if desired.

TASTY SALAD WITH GRILLED CHICKEN

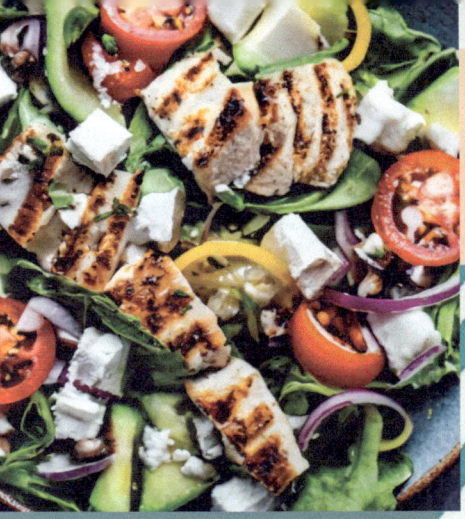

COOKING PROCESS:

In a bowl, whisk together 2 tablespoons of olive oil, minced garlic, dried oregano, salt, and black pepper.
Place the chicken breasts in a resealable plastic bag and pour the marinade over them.
Seal the bag and massage the marinade into the chicken.
Refrigerate for at least 30 minutes to marinate.
Preheat your grill to medium-high heat. Remove the chicken from the marinade and grill for about 6-7 minutes per side, or until the chicken is cooked through and has nice grill marks.
The internal temperature should reach 165°F (74°C).
Once cooked, remove the chicken from the grill, let it rest for a few minutes, then slice it into strips.
In a large salad bowl, combine the chopped romaine lettuce, cherry tomatoes, diced cucumber, thinly sliced red onion, Kalamata olives, crumbled feta cheese, and chopped fresh parsley.
In a small bowl, whisk together 1/4 cup extra-virgin olive oil, 2 tablespoons red wine vinegar, minced garlic, dried oregano, salt, and black pepper to taste.
Drizzle the Greek dressing over the salad ingredients.
Toss the salad gently to evenly coat everything with the dressing.
Arrange the sliced grilled chicken on top of the salad.
Serve the Greek Salad with Grilled Chicken immediately as a hearty and satisfying meal.

INGREDIENTS:

For the Grilled Chicken:

- 4 boneless, skinless chicken breasts
- 2 tablespoons olive oil
- 2 cloves garlic
- 1 teaspoon dried oregano
- Salt and black pepper to taste

For the Salad:

- 4 cups chopped romaine lettuce
- 1 cup cherry tomatoes
- 1 cucumber
- 1 red onion
- 1/2 cup Kalamata olives pitted
- 1/2 cup crumbled feta cheese
- 1/4 cup fresh parsley leaves

For the Greek Dressing:

- 1/4 cup extra-virgin olive oil
- 2 tablespoons red wine vinegar
- 1 clove garlic
- 1 teaspoon dried oregano
- Salt and black pepper to taste

MEDITERRANEAN WHOLE GRAIN BREAD

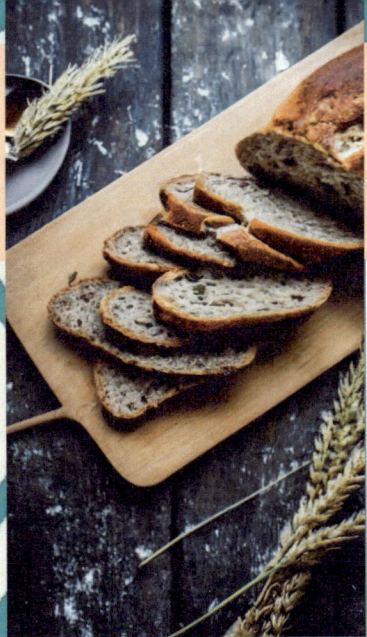

INGREDIENTS:

- 3 cups whole wheat flour
- 1 cup all-purpose flour
- 1 packet (2 1/4 teaspoon) active dry yeast
- 1 1/2 cups warm water
- 2 tablespoons extra virgin olive oil
- 1 teaspoon salt

COOKING PROCESS:

Activate the Yeast:
In a small bowl, combine the warm water and yeast. Let it sit for about 5-10 minutes until it becomes frothy. This indicates that the yeast is activated.

Mix the Flours:
In a large mixing bowl, combine the whole wheat flour and all-purpose flour.

Add Olive Oil and Salt:
Pour the activated yeast mixture into the bowl with the flour. Add the extra virgin olive oil and salt.

Knead the Dough:
Mix everything together to form a sticky dough. Turn the dough out onto a lightly floured surface and knead it for about 8-10 minutes until it becomes smooth and elastic. You can add a bit more flour if the dough is too sticky.

First Rise:
Place the dough in a greased bowl, cover it with a clean kitchen towel, and let it rise in a warm place for about 1-2 hours, or until it has doubled in size.

Punch Down and Shape:
Once the dough has risen, punch it down to release any excess air. Shape it into a round or oval loaf.

Second Rise:
Place the shaped dough onto a baking sheet lined with parchment paper. Cover it again and let it rise for another 30-45 minutes.

Preheat the Oven:
Preheat your oven to 375°F (190°C).

Bake:
Optionally, you can score the top of the bread with a sharp knife. Bake the bread in the preheated oven for about 30-35 minutes or until the crust is golden brown, and the bread sounds hollow when tapped on the bottom.

Cool:
Remove the bread from the oven and let it cool on a wire rack.

Slice and Serve:
Once the Mediterranean whole grain bread has cooled, slice it and serve it as part of a delicious meal, paired with olive oil, olives, and fresh vegetables, typical of Mediterranean cuisine.

SARDINIAN PANE CARASAU (SARDINIAN FLATBREAD)

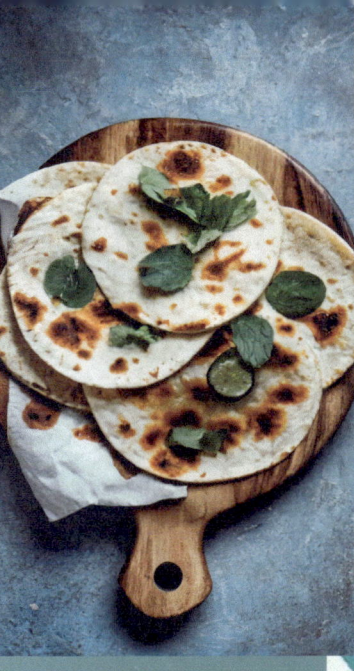

COOKING PROCESS:

Mix the Flours and Salt:
In a large mixing bowl, combine the semolina flour, all-purpose flour, and salt.

Add Warm Water:
Gradually add the warm water while stirring with a wooden spoon or your hands. Mix until a dough forms.

Knead the Dough:
Turn the dough out onto a clean, floured surface. Knead it for about 10-15 minutes until it becomes smooth and elastic. You may need to sprinkle a bit more flour if the dough is too sticky.

Divide the Dough:
Divide the dough into small, golf ball-sized portions. You should get approximately 8-10 portions.

Roll Out the Dough:
Take one portion of dough and roll it out as thinly as possible on a floured surface. Aim for a nearly paper-thin sheet, but it should still hold together.

Heat a Griddle or Skillet:
Preheat a dry griddle or non-stick skillet over medium-high heat.

Cook the Flatbread:
Place the rolled-out dough onto the hot griddle or skillet. Cook for about 1-2 minutes on each side or until it puffs up and gets lightly golden brown spots. You may need to press down gently with a spatula to encourage puffing.

Repeat:
Repeat the process with the remaining portions of dough.

Cool and Store:
Let the Pane Carasau cool completely on a wire rack. Once cooled, it can be stored in an airtight container for several weeks.

Serve: Pane Carasau is typically served as a crispy snack or accompaniment to other dishes. It can be enjoyed with toppings like fresh tomatoes, olive oil, and herbs, or used as a base for various toppings and spreads.

INGREDIENTS:

- 2 cups semolina flour
- 1 cup all-purpose flour
- 1 teaspoon salt
- 1 cup warm water

OKINAWAN SWEET POTATO BREAD

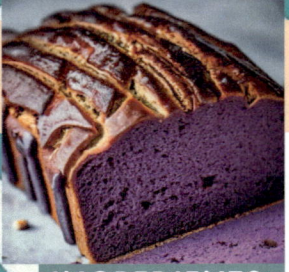

INGREDIENTS:
- 2 cups mashed Okinawan sweet potatoes
- 1/2 cup honey
- 1/4 cup coconut oil
- 2 eggs
- 1 1/2 cups all-purpose flour
- 1 tsp baking powder
- 1/2 tsp baking soda
- 1/2 tsp salt
- 1/2 tsp ground cinnamon
- 1/4 tsp ground nutmeg
- 1/4 cup walnuts

COOKING PROCESS:

Prepare Sweet Potatoes: Wash and peel potatoes. Cut them into small cubes and steam or boil until they are soft and easily mashable. Mash them in a bowl and let them cool to room temperature.

Preheat the Oven: Preheat your oven to 350°F (175°C). Grease and flour a loaf pan.

Combine Wet Ingredients: In a separate large mixing bowl, whisk together the honey, melted coconut oil, eggs, and mashed sweet potatoes until well combined.

Combine Dry Ingredients: In another bowl, sift together the all-purpose flour, baking powder, baking soda, salt, ground cinnamon, and ground nutmeg.

Combine Wet and Dry Mixtures: Gradually add the dry ingredients to the wet mixture, stirring until just combined. Be careful not to overmix; you want a slightly lumpy batter. If you're using chopped walnuts, fold them into the batter.

Fill the Loaf Pan: Pour the batter into the greased and floured loaf pan.

Bake: Place the loaf pan in the preheated oven and bake for about 45-55 minutes, or until a toothpick or cake tester inserted into the center comes out clean.

Cool: Remove the bread from the oven and let it cool in the pan for about 10 minutes. Then, transfer it to a wire rack to cool completely.

DELICIOUS WHOLE WHEAT PITA BREAD

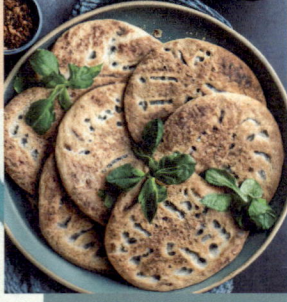

- 2 cups whole wheat flour
- 1 cup all-purpose flour
- 1 packet (2 1/4 teaspoon) active dry yeast
- 1 1/4 cups warm water
- 1 tsp salt
- 1 tsp sugar
- 2 tbsp olive oil

Activate the Yeast: In a small bowl, combine warm water, sugar, and yeast. Stir gently and let it sit for about 5-10 minutes, or until it becomes frothy. This indicates that the yeast is activated.

Prepare the Dough: In a large mixing bowl, combine the whole wheat flour and all-purpose flour. Add the salt and mix well.

Add Yeast Mixture: Pour the activated yeast mixture into the flour mixture. Add the olive oil.

Knead the Dough: Mix everything together until it forms a rough dough. Turn it out onto a floured surface and knead for about 5-7 minutes until the dough becomes smooth and elastic. You can add a bit more flour if it's too sticky.

Let the Dough Rise: Place the dough in a lightly oiled bowl, cover it with a clean kitchen towel, and let it rise in a warm, draft-free place for about 1 hour or until it has doubled in size.

Preheat the Oven: Preheat your oven to 475°F (245°C). Place a baking sheet or a pizza stone in the oven while it preheats.

Divide the Dough: Punch down the risen dough and divide it into 8 equal portions. Roll each portion into a ball.

Roll Out: On a floured surface, roll each dough ball into a thin circle, about 1/8-inch thick. You can use a rolling pin to achieve this.

Bake: Carefully place the rolled-out pitas onto the preheated baking sheet or pizza stone. Bake for about 2-3 minutes on each side, or until they puff up and turn golden brown.

REGIONAL MOCHI BREAD

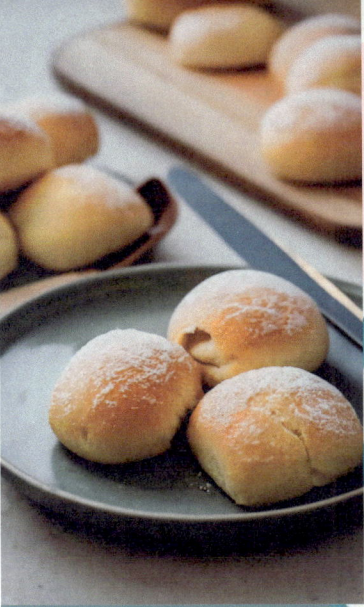

COOKING PROCESS:

Preheat the Oven:
Preheat your oven to 350°F (175°C).
Grease and flour a baking dish or a muffin tin.

Melt the Butter:
In a microwave-safe bowl or on the stovetop, melt the unsalted butter.

Mix Dry Ingredients:
In a separate bowl, combine the glutinous rice flour (mochiko) and baking powder.

Combine Wet Ingredients:
In a large mixing bowl, whisk together the melted butter, sugar, milk, sweetened condensed milk, and vanilla extract until well combined.

Add Eggs:
Beat the eggs and add them to the wet mixture. Mix thoroughly.

Mix Dry and Wet Ingredients:
Gradually add the dry ingredients to the wet mixture, stirring until you have a smooth batter.
If you're adding grated cheese, fold it into the batter.

Pour into Baking Dish:
Pour the batter into the greased and floured baking dish or muffin tin.

Bake:
Place it in the preheated oven and bake for approximately 25-30 minutes for a baking dish or 15-20 minutes for muffin-sized portions, or until the bread turns golden brown and a toothpick inserted into the center comes out clean.

Cool and Serve:
Remove the bread from the oven and let it cool for a few minutes.
Cut it into squares or serve the muffin-sized portions.
Japanese Mochi Bread is delicious when enjoyed warm.

INGREDIENTS:

- 1 cup glutinous rice flour (mochiko)
- 1/4 cup sugar
- 1/2 cup milk
- 1/4 cup unsalted butter
- 1/2 cup grated cheese (optional)
- 1/4 cup sweetened condensed milk
- 2 eggs
- 1 teaspoon baking powder
- 1/2 teaspoon vanilla extract

Side Dishes that Nourish

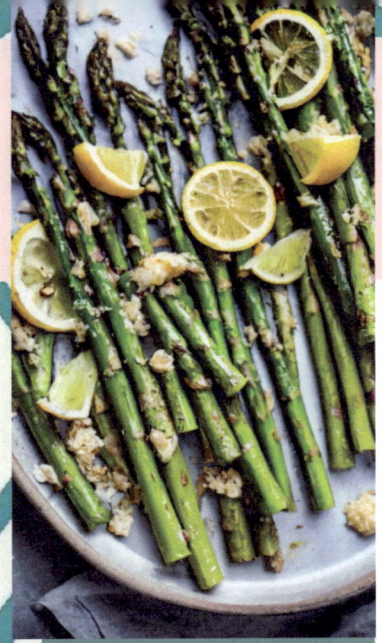

ROASTED ASPARAGUS WITH LEMON AND PARMESAN

INGREDIENTS:

- 1 bunch of fresh asparagus spears (about 1 pound)
- 2 tablespoons extra-virgin olive oil
- Zest of 1 lemon
- 2 tablespoons fresh lemon juice (about 1 lemon)
- 1/4 cup grated Parmesan cheese
- Salt and pepper, to taste

COOKING PROCESS:

Preheat your oven to 425°F (220°C).

Prepare the Asparagus:
Wash the asparagus spears and pat them dry with a clean kitchen towel.
Trim off the tough, woody ends of the asparagus. You can do this by holding each spear near the bottom and snapping off the tough part; it will naturally break at the right spot.

Arrange on a Baking Sheet:
Place the trimmed asparagus spears on a baking sheet in a single layer.

Season with Olive Oil:
Drizzle the asparagus olive oil. Season the asparagus with salt and pepper to taste.

Toss and Coat:
Gently toss the asparagus on the baking sheet to ensure that the spears are evenly coated with the olive oil, salt, and pepper.

Roast in the Oven:
Roast the asparagus in the preheated oven for about 10-15 minutes, or until they become tender and slightly browned. The exact cooking time may vary depending on the thickness of the asparagus, so keep an eye on them.

Prepare the Lemon and Parmesan Topping:
While the asparagus is roasting, prepare the lemon and Parmesan topping.
In a small bowl, combine the lemon zest, fresh lemon juice, and grated Parmesan cheese. Mix well to create the topping.

Finish and Serve:
Once the asparagus is done roasting, remove them from the oven.
Transfer the roasted asparagus to a serving platter.

Drizzle with Lemon and Parmesan:
Drizzle the lemon and Parmesan topping over the hot roasted asparagus while they are still on the serving platter.

Serve Immediately:
Serve the Roasted Asparagus with Lemon and Parmesan immediately, while it's still warm.

SWEET POTATO AND CHICKPEA PATTIES

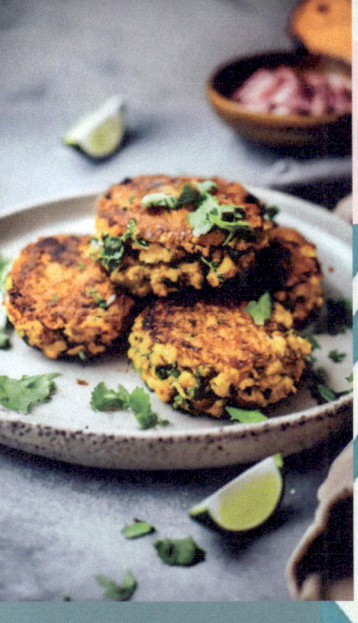

COOKING PROCESS:

Prepare Sweet Potatoes:
Peel and dice the sweet potatoes into small pieces.
Place the diced sweet potatoes in a pot of boiling water and cook until they are tender, which should take about 10-15 minutes.
Once cooked, drain the sweet potatoes and let them cool slightly.

Mash the Sweet Potatoes:
In a mixing bowl, mash the cooked sweet potatoes until they are smooth and free from lumps.

Prepare the Chickpeas:
In a food processor, combine the drained and rinsed chickpeas, breadcrumbs, grated Parmesan cheese, chopped fresh cilantro or parsley, ground cumin, smoked paprika, garlic powder, salt, and pepper.
Pulse the ingredients until the chickpeas are finely chopped and the mixture holds together.

Combine Sweet Potatoes and Chickpea Mixture:
Transfer the mashed sweet potatoes to the chickpea mixture in the food processor.
Pulse again to combine the ingredients until you have a uniform mixture.

Form Patties:
Divide the mixture into 8 portions and shape them into patties, similar to the size of burgers.

Cook the Patties:
In a skillet, heat a drizzle of olive oil over medium heat.
Once the oil is hot, add the sweet potato and chickpea patties to the skillet.
Cook the patties for about 3-4 minutes on each side or until they are golden brown and cooked through.
You may need to work in batches depending on the size of your skillet.

Serve:
Once cooked, transfer the Sweet Potato and Chickpea Patties to a serving platter or individual plates.
You can serve them with a side of fresh salad, yogurt-based sauce, or tahini sauce if desired.

INGREDIENTS:

- 2 medium-sized sweet potatoes
- 1 can (15 ounces) of chickpeas
- 1/2 cup breadcrumbs (you can use whole-grain breadcrumbs for a healthier option)
- 1/4 cup grated Parmesan cheese
- 1/4 cup fresh cilantro or parsley
- 1 teaspoon ground cumin
- 1 teaspoon smoked paprika
- 1/2 teaspoon garlic powder
- Salt and pepper, to taste
- Olive oil (for frying)

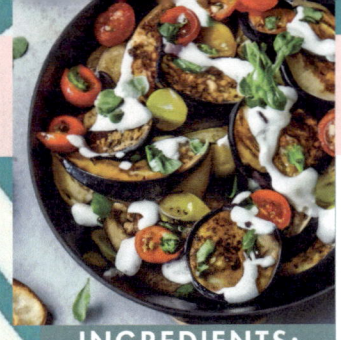

MEDITERRANEAN ROASTED EGGPLANT

INGREDIENTS:
- 2 medium-sized eggplants
- 1/4 cup extra-virgin olive oil
- 3 cloves garlic
- 1 tsp dried oregano
- 1 tsp dried basil
- 1/2 tsp dried thyme
- Salt and black pepper
- 1/4 cup fresh parsley (for garnish)
- Crumbled feta cheese for garnish (optional)

COOKING PROCESS:
Begin by washing and drying the eggplants. Cut off and discard the stem ends. Then, slice the eggplants into rounds or cubes, depending on your preference. You can choose to leave the skin on or peel it, depending on your texture preference.

In a small bowl, combine olive oil, minced garlic, dried oregano, dried basil, dried thyme, and salt and black pepper to taste. Mix these ingredients to create a flavorful marinade.

Place the sliced or cubed eggplants in a large mixing bowl. Pour the olive oil and herb mixture over the eggplants and toss them to coat them evenly.

Arrange the seasoned eggplants in a single layer on a baking sheet or roasting pan.

Roast the eggplants in the preheated oven for about 20-25 minutes or until they are tender and have a golden brown color. Be sure to flip them halfway through the roasting time for even cooking.

Serve hot, optionally, garnish the dish with chopped fresh parsley and crumbled feta cheese for added flavor and freshness.

LENTIL AND VEGETABLE STEW

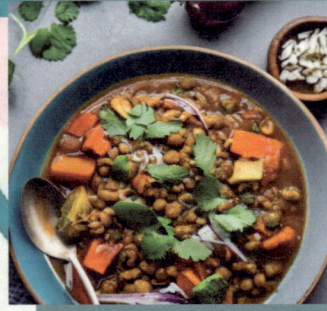

- 1 cup dried green or brown lentils
- 2 carrots
- 2 celery stalks
- 1 onion
- 2 cloves garlic
- 1 can (15 oz) tomatoes
- 4 cups vegetable broth
- 2 bay leaves
- 1 tsp dried thyme
- Salt and pepper
- Olive oil
- Fresh parsley (for garnish)

Start by rinsing dried green or brown lentils in a fine-mesh strainer under cold running water. Drain and set them aside.

In a large pot or Dutch oven, heat a bit of olive oil over medium heat. Add the chopped onion, diced carrots, and diced celery to the pot. Sauté the vegetables for about 5 minutes until they begin to soften.

Add the minced garlic to the sautéed vegetables and cook for an additional 30 seconds until fragrant. Stir in dried thyme and season with salt and pepper to taste.

Add the rinsed and drained lentils to the pot and stir to combine them with the vegetables. Pour in the entire can of diced tomatoes, including the juice, and stir again.

Pour vegetable broth into the pot. Enhance the flavor by incorporating bay leaves. Stir everything together to ensure all the ingredients are well combined. Bring the mixture to a boil over high heat. Once it's boiling, reduce the heat to low, cover the pot, and let the stew simmer for about 25-30 minutes, or until the lentils and vegetables are tender. Stir occasionally.

Taste and adjust the seasoning as needed, adding more salt and pepper if desired. Remove the bay leaves from the stew before serving.

WHOLESOME TZATZIKI AND VEGGIE PLATTER

COOKING PROCESS:

Grate the cucumber using a box grater or a food processor. Squeeze the grated cucumber in a clean kitchen towel or paper towel to remove excess moisture. In a mixing bowl, combine the Greek yogurt, minced garlic, grated and drained cucumber, chopped fresh dill, chopped fresh mint (if using), juice of 1 lemon, and olive oil.
Season the Tzatziki with salt and pepper to taste. Start with a pinch of each and adjust based on your preference. Mix all these ingredients thoroughly.
Arrange the freshly prepared Tzatziki in a shallow serving dish or on a platter.
Surround the Tzatziki with an array of fresh vegetables, such as cucumber slices, cherry tomatoes, baby carrots, bell pepper strips, and celery sticks. Sprinkle Kalamata olives and crumbled feta cheese over the Tzatziki for added flavor and texture.
Place whole-grain pita bread or pita chips alongside the platter for dipping and enjoying.

INGREDIENTS:
For the Tzatziki:
- 1 cup Greek yogurt
- 1 cucumber
- 2 cloves garlic
- 2 tbsp fresh dill
- 1 tbsp fresh mint
- Juice of 1 lemon
- 2 tbsp extra virgin olive oil
- Salt and pepper

For the Veggie Platter:
- An assortment: cucumber slices, cherry tomatoes, baby carrots, bell pepper strips, celery sticks
- Kalamata olives
- Feta chees
- Whole-grain pita bread or pita chips

ROASTED BEET AND GOAT CHEESE CROSTINI

Preheat your oven to 400°F (200°C). Place the diced beets on a baking sheet. Drizzle olive oil over the beets and season with salt and pepper to taste. Toss the beets to coat them evenly in the oil, salt, and pepper. Roast the beets in the preheated oven for approximately 25-30 minutes or until they are tender and slightly caramelized. Stir them once or twice during roasting for even cooking. Once roasted, remove the beets from the oven and let them cool slightly.
While the beets are roasting, prepare the crostini. Slice the baguette or French bread into thin rounds.
Place the bread rounds on a baking sheet and toast them in the oven at 400°F (200°C) for about 5-7 minutes or until they are crisp and slightly golden. Keep a close eye on them to avoid burning.
Once the roasted beets and crostini are ready, spread a generous amount of goat cheese onto each toasted bread round.
Top the goat cheese with a few pieces of roasted beets. You can press them gently into the cheese to help them adhere.
Sprinkle fresh thyme leaves over the beets for a burst of flavor and aroma. Drizzle honey lightly over each crostini for a touch of sweetness and elegance.

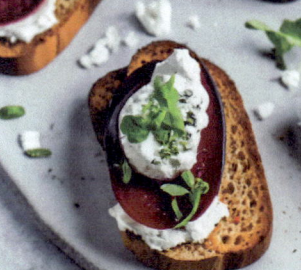

For the Roasted Beets:
- 4 small to medium sized beets
- 2 tablespoons extra virgin olive oil
- Salt and pepper, to taste

For the Crostini:
- 1 baguette or French bread
- 4 ounces goat cheese (chevre)
- Fresh thyme leaves, for garnish
- Honey, for drizzling

Side Dishes that Nourish

ROASTED RED PEPPER AND WALNUT DIP

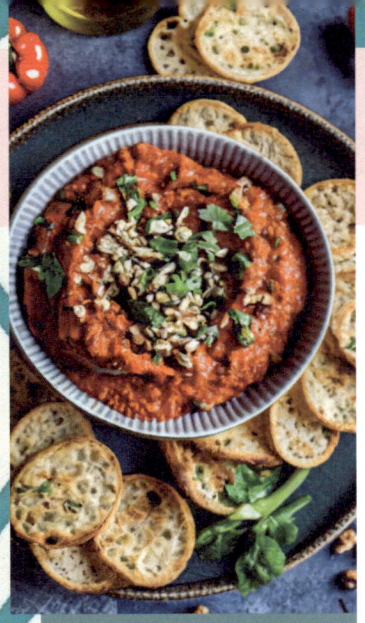

INGREDIENTS:

- 2 large red bell peppers
- 1 cup walnuts
- 2 cloves garlic
- 2 tablespoons extra virgin olive oil
- 2 tablespoons fresh lemon juice
- 1 teaspoon ground cumin
- 1/2 teaspoon paprika (smoked or regular)
- Salt and pepper, to taste
- Fresh parsley or mint leaves (for garnish)
- Whole-grain pita bread or pita chips (for serving)

COOKING PROCESS:

Preheat your oven to 425°F (220°C).
Place the red bell peppers directly on the oven rack or on a baking sheet lined with aluminum foil.
Roast the peppers for about 25-30 minutes, turning them occasionally with tongs, until the skin is charred and blistered.
Remove the roasted peppers from the oven and immediately place them in a heatproof bowl. Cover the bowl with plastic wrap or a clean kitchen towel and let them steam for about 10 minutes. This will make it easier to peel off the skin.
While the peppers are steaming, toast the walnuts.
Place the walnuts in a dry skillet over medium-low heat.
Toast them for about 3-5 minutes, stirring frequently, until they become fragrant and lightly golden. Be careful not to over-toast, as walnuts can burn quickly.
Set aside to cool.
After steaming, the roasted peppers should be cool enough to handle. Peel off the charred skin and remove the seeds. You can also rinse them under cold water to remove any remaining skin or seeds.
Cut the peeled and seeded peppers into strips.
In a food processor, combine the roasted red pepper strips, toasted walnuts, minced garlic, olive oil, fresh lemon juice, ground cumin, paprika, salt, and pepper.
Blend the ingredients until you achieve a smooth and creamy dip. If it's too thick, you can add a bit of water (1-2 tablespoons at a time) and blend until it reaches your desired texture.
Taste the dip and adjust the seasonings if necessary. You can add more lemon juice, garlic, cumin, or salt based on your preference.
Transfer the Roasted Red Pepper and Walnut Dip to a serving bowl or dish.
Garnish with fresh parsley or mint leaves for a burst of color and flavor.
Serve the dip with whole-grain pita bread or pita chips for dipping and enjoying.

Spinach and Feta Stuffed Mini Peppers

Cooking Process:

Wash and dry the mini bell peppers. Cut off the tops of each pepper and remove the seeds and membranes, creating little pepper cups.
In a mixing bowl, combine the finely chopped fresh spinach, crumbled feta cheese, ricotta cheese, minced garlic, grated Parmesan cheese, and red pepper flakes (if using). Season the filling mixture with salt and pepper to taste. Be mindful of the salt, as feta cheese can be salty.
Using a spoon, stuff each mini pepper with the spinach and cheese mixture. Press the filling down gently to ensure the peppers are well-filled.
Place the stuffed mini peppers on a baking sheet lined with parchment paper or lightly greased with olive oil.
Drizzle a bit of olive oil over the stuffed mini-peppers. This helps them roast and develop a nice texture.
Preheat your oven to 375°F (190°C). Roast the stuffed mini peppers in the preheated oven for approximately 20-25 minutes or until the peppers are tender and slightly blistered, and the filling is heated through.
Once cooked, transfer Peppers to a serving platter or individual plates.

Ingredients:
- 16-20 mini bell peppers (a mix of colors)
- 1 cup fresh spinach
- 1/2 cup crumbled feta cheese
- 1/4 cup ricotta cheese
- 2 cloves garlic
- 1/4 cup grated Parmesan cheese
- 1/4 tsp red pepper flakes (optional, for a hint of heat)
- Salt and pepper
- Olive oil (for drizzling)

Stuffed Mushrooms with Quinoa and Spinach

Start by cleaning the mushrooms. Gently wipe them with a damp cloth or paper towel to remove any dirt. Remove the stems from the mushrooms and set them aside.
In a skillet, heat olive oil over medium heat. Add the minced garlic and sauté for about 1 minute until fragrant. Add the chopped spinach to the skillet and sauté for another 2-3 minutes until it wilts. Season with a pinch of salt and pepper. In a mixing bowl, combine the cooked quinoa, sautéed spinach, cheese, and the sautéed garlic and spinach mixture. Mix well to create the filling.
Preheat your oven to 375°F (190°C). Place the cleaned mushrooms on a baking sheet or in a baking dish, cap side down. Fill each mushroom cap generously with the quinoa and spinach filling, pressing it down slightly.
In a small bowl, combine breadcrumbs with grated Parmesan cheese to create the topping mixture.
Sprinkle the breadcrumb and Parmesan topping mixture over each stuffed mushroom, pressing it gently to adhere. Bake the stuffed mushrooms in the preheated oven for approximately 20-25 minutes or until the mushrooms are tender and the topping is golden brown.
Once baked, remove the stuffed mushrooms from the oven and let them cool slightly. Garnish with freshly chopped parsley for a burst of color and flavor.

For the Stuffed Mushrooms:
- 16 large white or cremini mushrooms
- 1 cup cooked quinoa (about 1/2 cup uncooked quinoa)
- 1 cup fresh spinach
- 1/2 cup grated Parmesan cheese
- 2 cloves garlic
- 2 tbsp olive oil
- Salt and pepper

For the Topping:
- 1/4 cup breadcrumbs (or whole-grain)
- 2 tbsp grated Parmesan cheese
- Fresh parsley

SUNNY CAPRESE STUFFED PORTOBELLO MUSHROOMS

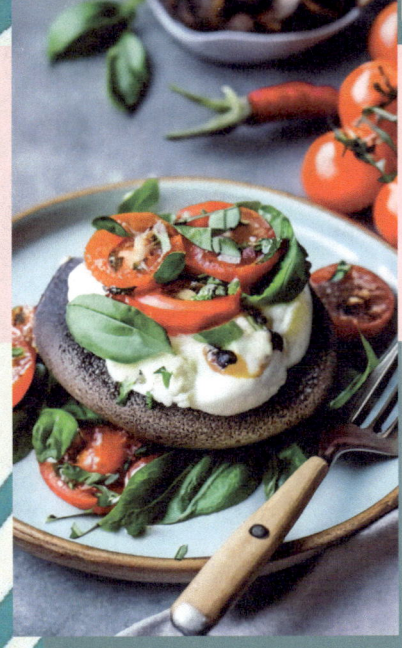

INGREDIENTS:

- 4 large Portobello mushrooms
- 2 tablespoons olive oil
- 2 cloves garlic
- Salt and black pepper to taste
- 1 cup cherry tomatoes
- 1 cup fresh mozzarella balls or mozzarella
- 1/4 cup fresh basil leaves
- Balsamic glaze for drizzling (optional)

COOKING PROCESS:

Preheat your oven to 425°F (220°C).
Clean the Portobello mushrooms by gently wiping them with a damp cloth.
Remove the stems and use a spoon to scrape out the gills to create space for the stuffing.
Place the cleaned Portobello mushrooms on a baking sheet.
Drizzle them with olive oil and minced garlic. Season with salt and black pepper to taste.
Make sure the mushrooms are well-coated.
Roast the mushrooms in the preheated oven for about 10-12 minutes, or until they start to soften.
While the mushrooms are roasting, prepare the Caprese filling.
In a bowl, combine the halved cherry tomatoes, fresh mozzarella balls or cubes, and torn basil leaves.
Toss gently to mix.
Once the mushrooms are done roasting, remove them from the oven.
Drain any excess liquid that may have accumulated inside the mushrooms.
Stuff each Portobello mushroom with the Caprese filling mixture, pressing it down gently to ensure they are well-filled.
Return the stuffed Portobello mushrooms to the oven and bake for an additional 10-15 minutes, or until the mushrooms are tender and the cheese is melted and bubbly.
Remove the stuffed mushrooms from the oven and let them cool slightly before serving.
Drizzle with balsamic glaze if desired.

Side Dishes that Nourish

QUINOA AND BLACK BEAN STUFFED PEPPERS

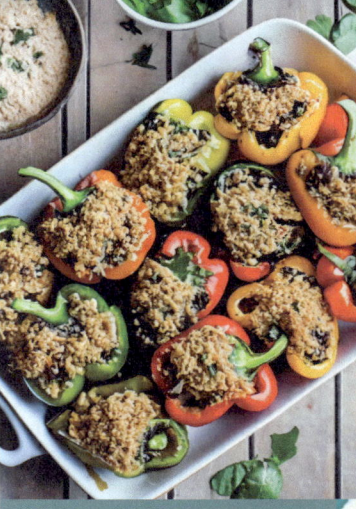

COOKING PROCESS:

Wash the bell peppers and cut off the tops. Remove the seeds and membranes to create pepper cups. Set aside.

In a medium saucepan, rinse the quinoa under cold water until the water runs clear. Combine the rinsed quinoa with vegetable broth or water.

Bring the mixture to a boil over medium-high heat. Once boiling, reduce the heat to low, cover, and simmer for about 15-20 minutes or until the quinoa is cooked and has absorbed the liquid.

Remove the quinoa from the heat and fluff it with a fork. Set aside.

In a large skillet, heat a drizzle of olive oil over medium heat.

Add the diced red onion and minced garlic to the skillet and sauté until they become fragrant and translucent.

Add the ground cumin, chili powder, smoked paprika, salt, and pepper to the skillet, and stir to coat the onions and garlic with the spices.

Open a can of black beans, drain, and rinse thoroughly. Stir in the black beans, corn kernels, and diced tomatoes. Cook for an additional 2-3 minutes until the mixture is heated through.

Transfer the cooked quinoa to the skillet with the bean and vegetable mixture.

Stir everything together until well combined. Taste and adjust the seasoning, if necessary.

Preheat your oven to 375°F (190°C). Carefully stuff each bell pepper with the quinoa and black bean mixture, pressing it down gently to ensure it's well packed.

Place the stuffed peppers in a baking dish.

Drizzle a little olive oil over the tops of the stuffed peppers. Cover the baking dish with aluminum foil.

Bake the stuffed peppers in the preheated oven for about 30-35 minutes, or until the peppers are tender and cooked to your liking.

If you like, you can remove the foil during the last 10 minutes of baking and sprinkle grated cheese on top of each stuffed pepper. Return them to the oven until the cheese is melted and bubbly.

Once cooked, remove Peppers from the oven.

Serve them hot, garnished with fresh herbs if desired.

INGREDIENTS:

- 4 large bell peppers (any color)
- 1 cup quinoa
- 2 cups vegetable broth or water
- 1 can (15 ounces) black beans
- 1 cup corn kernels (fresh, frozen, or canned)
- 1 cup diced tomatoes (canned or fresh)
- 1 cup diced red onion
- 2 cloves garlic
- 1 teaspoon ground cumin
- 1/2 teaspoon chili powder
- 1/2 teaspoon smoked paprika
- Salt and pepper, to taste
- Olive oil, for drizzling
- Grated cheese (optional, for topping)

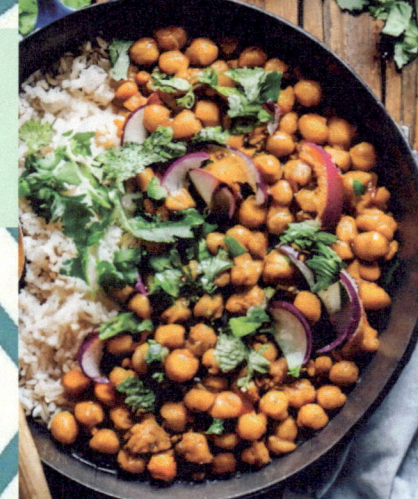

VEGAN TAGINE WITH CHICKPEAS

INGREDIENTS:

For the Chickpea Tagine:
- 2 tablespoons olive oil
- 1 large onion
- 3 cloves garlic
- 1 teaspoon ground cumin
- 1 teaspoon ground coriander
- 1 teaspoon ground paprika
- 1/2 teaspoon ground cinnamon
- 1/4 teaspoon ground ginger
- 1/4 teaspoon cayenne pepper (adjust to taste)
- 2 cans (15 ounces each) chickpeas, drained and rinsed
- 1 can (14.5 ounces) diced tomatoes
- 1 cup vegetable broth
- 1 cup carrots
- 1 cup bell peppers (red and green)
- 1 cup zucchini
- Salt and black pepper to taste
- Fresh cilantro or parsley for garnish

For Serving:
- Cooked couscous or ricetional)

COOKING PROCESS:

In a large tagine or a deep skillet with a lid, heat 2 tablespoons of olive oil over medium heat.
Add the finely chopped onion and minced garlic to the hot oil.
Saute for 3-4 minutes until the onion becomes translucent.
Stir in the ground cumin, ground coriander, ground paprika, ground cinnamon, ground ginger, and cayenne pepper.
Cook for another minute to toast the spices.
Add the drained chickpeas and diced tomatoes (with their juices) to the tagine.
Stir well to combine with the spices and onions.
Pour in the vegetable broth, and stir to combine.
Bring the mixture to a simmer.
Add the diced carrots, bell peppers, and zucchini to the tagine.
Stir to combine all the ingredients.
Season with salt and black pepper to taste.
Cover the tagine with a lid and reduce the heat to low. Let it simmer for 20-25 minutes, or until the vegetables are tender.
Taste the tagine and adjust the seasoning if needed.
You can add more salt, pepper, or spices to your liking.
Serve the Moroccan Chickpea Tagine hot, garnished with fresh cilantro or parsley.
Serve the tagine over cooked couscous or rice for a complete meal.

OKINAWAN STIR-FRIED VEGETABLES

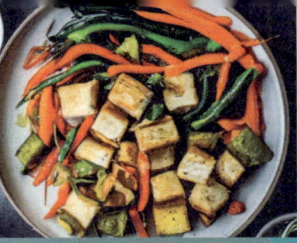

COOKING PROCESS:

Peel and cut the potatoes into thin slices or sticks. If you can't find Okinawan potatoes, regular sweet potatoes can be used as a substitute. Cut the long beans or green beans into 2-inch pieces. Julienne the carrots. Thinly slice the bell peppers. Cube the firm tofu.
Bring a pot of water to a boil and add the purple sweet potato slices. Blanch for about 2-3 minutes or until they are slightly tender. Drain and set aside.
In a large skillet or wok, heat the vegetable oil over medium-high heat. Add the minced garlic to the hot oil and stir-fry for about 30 seconds until fragrant.
Add the blanched potatoes, long beans, carrots, and bell peppers to the skillet. Stir-fry for about 5-7 minutes or until the vegetables start to soften but still have a crisp texture.
Add the cubed tofu to the skillet and gently mix it with the vegetables. Drizzle soy sauce (and oyster sauce if using) over the vegetables and tofu. Stir-fry for an additional 2-3 minutes, ensuring the sauce coats all the ingredients evenly.
Season with salt and pepper to taste. Garnish with fresh cilantro or parsley leaves.

INGREDIENTS:
- 2 cups Okinawan purple sweet potatoes
- 2 cups long beans or green beans
- 1 cup carrots
- 1 cup bell peppers (any color)
- 1 cup firm tofu
- 2 tbsp vegetable oil
- 2 cloves garlic
- 2 tbsp soy sauce (adjust to taste)
- 1 tbsp oyster sauce
- Salt and pepper
- Fresh cilantro or parsley leaves

FLAVORFUL LEMON AND GARLIC ROASTED CHICKEN

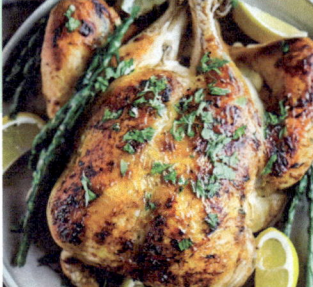

Preheat your oven to 375°F(190°C). Rinse the whole chicken under cold water and pat it dry with paper towels. Place the chicken in a roasting pan or a baking dish.
In a small bowl, combine the minced garlic, olive oil, dried oregano, dried thyme, dried rosemary, and the juice and zest of 1 lemon. Mix well to create the marinade.
Carefully lift the skin of the chicken, being careful not to tear it, and rub the marinade mixture under the skin and all over the chicken, including the cavity. Season the chicken with salt and black pepper, both inside and out.
Cut the remaining lemon into quarters and stuff them into the chicken's cavity. This will infuse the chicken with lemon flavor as it roasts.
Place the prepared chicken in the preheated oven and roast for approximately 1 hour and 15 minutes to 1 hour and 30 minutes, or until the chicken's internal temperature reaches 165°F(74°C) and the skin is golden brown and crispy. Baste the chicken with pan juices every 30 minutes.
Once the chicken is done, remove it from the oven and let it rest for about 10-15 minutes. This allows the juices to redistribute and keeps the meat tender.
Garnish with fresh rosemary sprigs and lemon slices if desired.

INGREDIENTS:
- 1 whole chicken (about 3-4 pounds)
- 2 lemons
- 4-6 cloves garlic
- 2 tbsp olive oil
- 1 tsp dried oregano
- 1 tsp dried thyme
- 1 tsp dried rosemary
- Salt and black pepper
- Fresh rosemary and lemon slices for garnish (optional)

Delectable Main Courses for Health

GRILLED CHICKEN WITH HERBED QUINOA

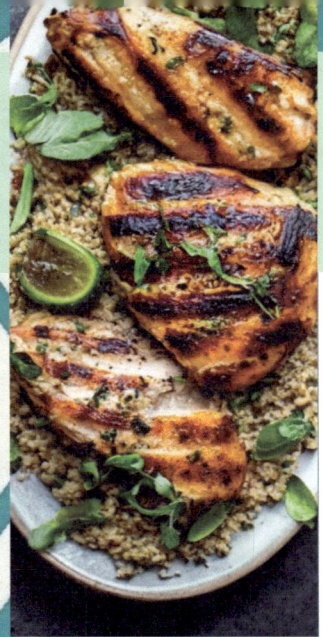

INGREDIENTS:

- 4 boneless, skinless chicken breasts
- 1 cup quinoa
- Fresh parsley, mint, and dill
- Zest of 1 lemon
- 2 cloves garlic
- Olive oil
- Salt and pepper to taste

COOKING PROCESS:

Rinse 1 cup of quinoa under cold running water in a fine-mesh strainer. In a medium saucepan, add the rinsed quinoa and 2 cups of water.
Bring the mixture to a boil over high heat.
Once boiling, reduce the heat to low, cover the saucepan, and let the quinoa simmer for 15-20 minutes, or until all the liquid is absorbed. Remove the saucepan from the heat and let it sit, covered, for an additional 5 minutes.
After resting, fluff the quinoa with a fork to separate the grains.
While the quinoa is still warm, add a generous handful of chopped fresh parsley, mint, and dill.
Mix in the zest of 1 lemon, minced garlic, a drizzle of olive oil, and season with salt and pepper to taste.
Toss everything together to evenly distribute the herbs and flavors. Set the herbed quinoa aside.
Preheat your grill to medium-high heat. Make sure it's clean and well-oiled to prevent sticking.
Season each of the chicken breasts with olive oil, lemon zest, minced garlic, and a generous sprinkle of salt and pepper.
Gently rub the seasonings into the chicken breasts to ensure they're evenly coated.
Place the seasoned chicken breasts on the preheated grill.
Grill for approximately 6-8 minutes on each side, or until the chicken is cooked through and no longer pink in the center.
Use a meat thermometer to check the internal temperature, which should reach 165°F (74°C).
Cooking times may vary depending on the thickness of the chicken breasts, so adjust as needed.
Once the chicken is cooked to perfection, remove it from the grill.
Let the grilled chicken rest for a few minutes to allow the juices to redistribute.
To serve, plate each chicken breast on a bed of herbed quinoa, garnishing with additional fresh herbs if desired.

Delectable Main Courses for Health

OSSO BUCO (VEAL OR BEEF SHANK STEW)

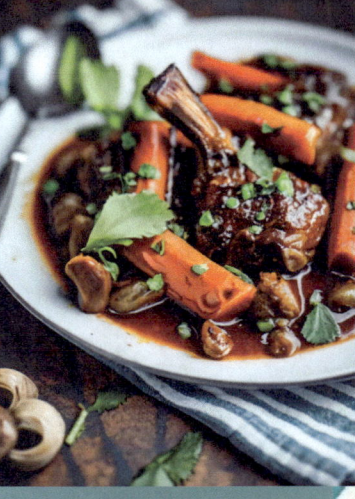

COOKING PROCESS:

Begin by slicing the veal or beef shanks, each about 1.5 inches thick.
Then, seasoning the veal or beef shanks generously with salt and freshly ground black pepper. Dredge them in all-purpose flour, shaking off any excess.
In a large, heavy-bottomed skillet or Dutch oven, heat the olive oil over medium-high heat. Add the shanks and sear them until they are browned on all sides, about 5 minutes per side. Transfer the seared shanks to a plate and set them aside.
In the same skillet or Dutch oven, add the finely chopped onion, carrots, celery, and minced garlic. Cook, stirring frequently, until the vegetables are softened and the onion is translucent about 5 minutes.
Pour in the dry white wine and allow it to simmer for a few minutes, scraping up any browned bits from the bottom of the pan with a wooden spoon.
Return the seared shanks to the pan and add the diced tomatoes, beef or vegetable broth, fresh rosemary, fresh thyme, and lemon zest. Stir everything together.
Bring the mixture to a gentle simmer, then reduce the heat to low. Cover the pan with a lid and let it simmer for about 2 to 2.5 hours, or until the meat is tender and easily pulls away from the bone. Check occasionally and add more broth or water if needed to keep the shanks moist.
While the stew is simmering, you can prepare the gremolata, if desired. In a small bowl, combine the finely chopped fresh parsley, lemon zest, and minced garlic. This mixture will be used as a garnish for the Osso Buco.
Once the meat is tender, remove the shanks from the pan and place them on a serving platter.
To serve, spoon the rich, flavorful sauce over the shanks and garnish with the gremolata.
Osso Buco is traditionally served with risotto or polenta, but you can also pair it with mashed potatoes or crusty bread to soak up the delicious sauce.

INGREDIENTS:

- 4 veal or beef shanks
- Salt and freshly ground black pepper, to taste
- 1/2 cup all-purpose flour, for dredging
- 3 tablespoons olive oil
- 1 onion
- 2 carrots
- 2 celery stalks
- 4 cloves garlic
- 1 cup dry white wine
- 1 can (14 ounces) diced tomatoes
- 1 cup beef or vegetable broth
- 2 sprigs fresh rosemary
- 2 sprigs fresh thyme
- Zest of 1 lemon

Gremolata (optional garnish):

- 2 tablespoons fresh parsley
- Zest of 1 lemon
- 2 cloves garlic

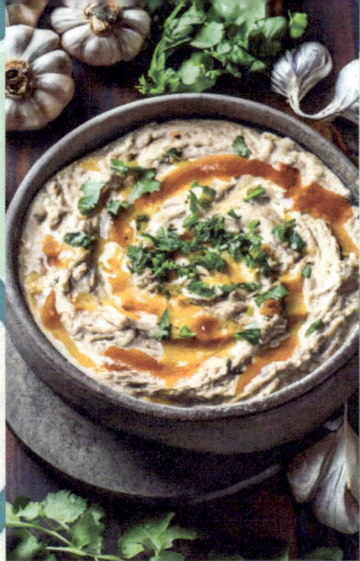

ROASTED GARLIC AND WHITE BEAN DIP

INGREDIENTS:

- 2 cans (15 ounces each) of white beans (such as cannellini or Great Northern)
- 1 whole head of garlic
- 2 tablespoons extra- virgin olive oil
- 2 tablespoons fresh lemon juice (about 1 lemon)
- 2 tablespoons tahini (sesame paste)
- 1/4 teaspoon ground cumin
- Salt and pepper, to taste
- Fresh parsley or chives, for garnish (optional)
- Vegetables, pita bread, or crackers for dipping

COOKING PROCESS:

Preheat your oven to 400°F (200°C).
Cut off the top quarter of the head of garlic to expose the cloves.
Drizzle the exposed garlic cloves with a bit of olive oil and wrap the entire head of garlic in aluminum foil.
Roast the garlic in the preheated oven for about 35-45 minutes, or until the cloves are soft and golden brown.
Remove the roasted garlic from the oven and let it cool slightly.
Once cool enough to handle, squeeze the roasted garlic cloves out of their skins into a small bowl.
In a food processor or blender, combine the drained and rinsed white beans, roasted garlic cloves, 2 tablespoons of extra-virgin olive oil, fresh lemon juice, tahini, ground cumin, salt, and pepper.
Blend the mixture until it is completely smooth and creamy. You may need to scrape down the sides of the processor or blender and blend again to ensure there are no lumps.
Taste the dip and adjust the seasoning as needed. You can add more lemon juice, salt, or pepper to suit your taste.
Transfer the Roasted Garlic and White Bean Dip to a serving bowl.
Drizzle a bit of extra-virgin olive oil over the top for garnish.
If desired, sprinkle fresh parsley or chives over the dip for a pop of color and added flavor.
Arrange an assortment of sliced vegetables, pita bread, or crackers around the dip for dipping.

QUINOA-STUFFED BELL PEPPERS

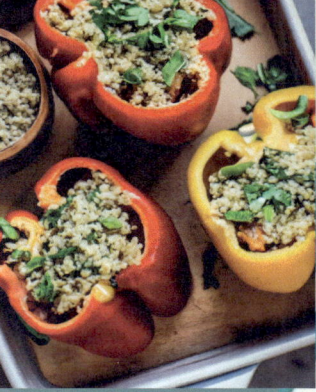

COOKING PROCESS:

Preheat your oven to 375°F (190°C). Cut the tops off the bell peppers and remove the seeds and membranes from inside. Rinse the peppers under cold water and set them aside to drain.

Rinse quinoa under cold running water in a fine-mesh strainer. In a medium saucepan, add the rinsed quinoa and 2 cups of water. Bring the mixture to a boil over high heat. Once boiling, reduce the heat to low, cover the saucepan, and let the quinoa simmer for 15-20 minutes, or until all the liquid is absorbed. Remove the saucepan from the heat and let it sit, covered, for an additional 5 minutes. After resting, fluff the quinoa with a fork to separate the grains.

In a large mixing bowl, combine the cooked quinoa, can drained and rinsed black beans, corn kernels, diced tomatoes, and chopped onion. Season the mixture with cumin and chili powder.

Carefully stuff each bell pepper with the quinoa and vegetable mixture. Fill them to the top without over-packing.

Place peppers in a baking dish, standing upright. Cover the dish with aluminum foil to trap steam and moisture. Bake in the preheated oven for 30-35 minutes or until the peppers are tender when pierced with a fork.

Remove peppers from the oven and let them cool slightly. Serve them with your choice of salsa, either store-bought or homemade, drizzled on top for added flavor.

INGREDIENTS:

- 4 large bell peppers (any color)
- 1 cup quinoa
- 1 can (15 oz) black beans
- 1 cup corn kernels (fresh or frozen)
- 2 tomatoes
- 1 onion
- 2 teaspoons cumin
- 1 teaspoon chili powder
- Salsa (store-bought or homemade)

ZUCCHINI AND TOMATO SKEWERS

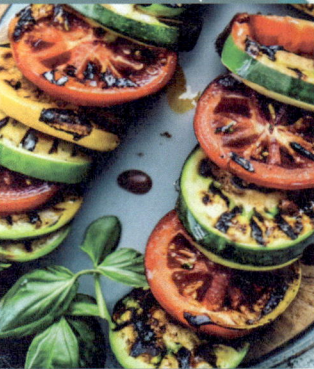

In a mixing bowl, combine oil, minced garlic, chopped fresh basil, chopped fresh oregano, salt, and pepper. Mix well to create the marinade.

Preheat your grill to medium-high heat. If using wooden skewers, soak them in water for at least 30 minutes to prevent burning.

Wash the zucchini and cherry tomatoes. Cut the zucchini into 1-inch thick rounds. Thread the zucchini rounds and cherry tomatoes alternately onto the skewers, creating a colorful pattern.

Brush the marinade over the zucchini and tomato skewers, ensuring that they are well-coated.

Place the skewers on the preheated grill. Grill for approximately 4-5 minutes on each side, or until the vegetables are tender and have grill marks. Be sure to monitor them closely to prevent overcooking.

Once the skewers are cooked to your liking, remove them from the grill and transfer them to a serving platter.

- 2 medium zucchini
- 2 cups cherry tomatoes
- 1/4 cup extra-virgin olive oil
- 2 cloves garlic
- 1 tablespoon fresh basil
- 1 tablespoon fresh oregano
- Salt and pepper
- Wooden skewers

TOFU AND VEGETABLE STIR-FRY

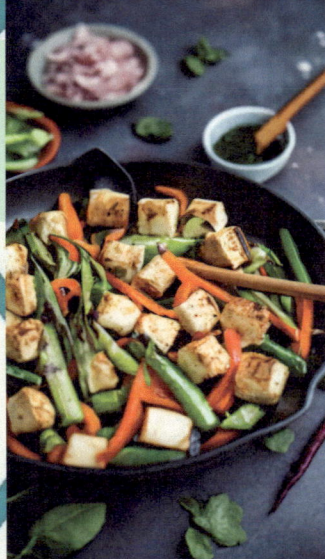

INGREDIENTS:

- 1 block of tofu
- Assorted vegetables:
    broccoli
    bell peppers
    snap peas
    carrots
- 2 cloves garlic
- 2 tablespoons soy sauce
- 1 tablespoon sesame oil
- 1 tablespoon cornstarch
- Olive oil
- Cooked rice

COOKING PROCESS:

Start by pressing the tofu to remove excess moisture. Place the block of tofu on a clean kitchen towel or paper towel. Cover it with more towels and place a heavy object on top (like a cast iron skillet). Allow it to press for about 15-20 minutes. This helps the tofu absorb flavors better and become firmer.
After pressing, cut the tofu into bite-sized cubes.
Wash and chop your choice of assorted vegetables. Common choices include broccoli florets, bell peppers (sliced), snap peas, and carrots (sliced or julienned). Keep the vegetables ready for stir-frying.
In a small bowl, whisk together soy sauce, sesame oil, and cornstarch. This will be your stir-fry sauce.
Heat a wok or a large skillet over medium-high heat. Add a tablespoon of olive oil to the hot pan.
Carefully add the cubed tofu to the hot oil. Stir-fry the tofu until it turns golden brown and slightly crispy on all sides. This can take about 5-7 minutes.
Once done, remove the tofu from the pan and set it aside.
In the same pan, add more olive oil if needed.
Add the minced garlic to the hot oil and sauté for about 30 seconds until it becomes fragrant.
Add the chopped vegetables to the pan.
Stir-fry the vegetables for approximately 3-4 minutes or until they become tender-crisp. You want them to retain some crunch.
Return the cooked tofu to the pan with the sautéed vegetables.
Pour the prepared stir-fry sauce (soy sauce, sesame oil, and cornstarch mixture) over the tofu and vegetables. Stir everything together to evenly coat the tofu and vegetables with the sauce.
Continue stir-frying for an additional 2 minutes to heat the tofu and meld the flavors.
Taste the stir-fry and adjust the seasoning if necessary, adding more soy sauce or sesame oil as desired.
Serve the tofu and vegetable stir-fried hot cooked rice of your choice (white rice, brown rice, or jasmine rice).

GRILLED EGGPLANT AND ZUCCHINI RATATOUILLE

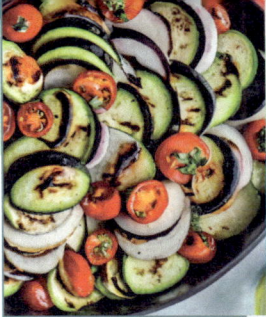

COOKING PROCESS:

Preheat your grill to medium-high heat. Make sure it's clean and well-oiled to prevent sticking.
Slice the eggplant, zucchini, tomatoes, and red bell pepper into rounds or slices. You want them to be of similar thickness for even cooking. Chop the onion and mince the garlic. Gather fresh basil, thyme, and oregano for seasoning.
In a large mixing bowl, combine all the sliced vegetables (eggplant, zucchini, tomatoes, and red bell pepper). Drizzle olive oil over the vegetables and season them generously with salt, pepper, and minced garlic. Toss the vegetables to ensure they are well-coated with the oil and seasonings.
Place the seasoned vegetable slices on the preheated grill grates. Grill the vegetables until they have grill marks and are tender. This usually takes about 3-4 minutes per side, but times may vary depending on your grill's heat.
As the vegetables finish grilling, remove them from the grill and arrange them in a casserole dish, layering them. You can layer them in any order you like.
Drizzle a bit more olive oil over the grilled vegetables. Season them with additional fresh herbs (basil, thyme, and oregano) to taste. Season with extra salt and pepper if desired.
Preheat your oven to 350°F(175°C). Place the casserole dish with the grilled vegetables in the oven. Bake for 15-20 minutes to melt the flavors and ensure all the vegetables are tender.

INGREDIENTS:
- 1 eggplant
- 2 zucchini
- 2 tomatoes
- 1 red bell pepper
- 1 onion
- 2 cloves garlic
- Fresh basil, thyme and oregano
- Olive oil
- Salt and pepper to taste

WHOLE WHEAT PASTA PRIMAVERA

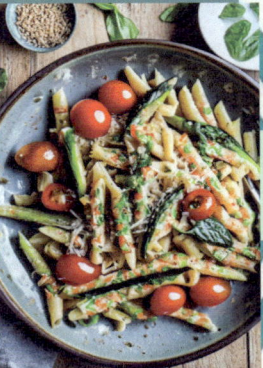

In a large pot, bring water to a boil. Add a pinch of salt to the boiling water. Add whole wheat pasta to the boiling water. Cook the pasta according to the package instructions until it's al dente (firm to the bite). Once cooked, drain the pasta in a colander and set it aside. Do not rinse it.
Wash and chop the assorted seasonal vegetables of your choice. Popular choices include zucchini, cherry tomatoes, and asparagus, but feel free to use any vegetables you prefer. Cut them into bite-sized pieces for easy mixing.
In a large skillet, heat olive oil over medium heat. Add minced garlic to the hot oil and sauté for about 30 seconds until it becomes fragrant. Add the chopped seasonal vegetables to the skillet. Sauté the vegetables for approximately 3-4 minutes or until they start to soften and become slightly tender. Season the vegetables with a pinch of salt and pepper to taste.
Add the cooked whole wheat pasta to the skillet with the sautéed vegetables. Gently toss the pasta and vegetables together to mix them evenly. The pasta will absorb some of the flavors from the vegetables and garlic.
Toss in a handful of freshly chopped basil and parsley to add a burst of fresh flavor to the dish. Adjust the quantity of herbs to your preference.
If desired, top each serving with Parmesan for extra flavor.

- 8 oz whole wheat pasta (penne or spaghetti)
- Assorted seasonal vegetables (zucchini, cherry tomatoes, asparagus)
- 2 cloves garlic
- Olive oil
- Fresh basil and parsley
- Salt and pepper
- Grated Parmesan cheese

Delectable Main Courses for Health

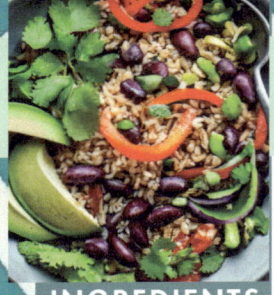

BROWN RICE AND BLACK BEAN BOWL

INGREDIENTS:

- 2 cups cooked brown rice
- 1 can (15 oz) black beans
- 1 cup corn kernels (fresh or frozen)
- 2 avocados
- 1 red onion
- Fresh cilantro
- Lime juice
- Ground cumin
- Salt and pepper

COOKING PROCESS:

If you haven't already cooked the brown rice, follow the package instructions to prepare the required amount of cooked brown rice. Set it aside.

Drain and rinse a can of black beans under cold running water. This helps remove excess sodium and ensures they're clean.

If you're using fresh corn, you can cook it by either boiling or grilling. Once cooked, cut the kernels off the cob.

Dice avocados and finely chopped red onion. Gather a handful of fresh cilantro and chop it coarsely. You can use as much cilantro as you prefer, depending on your taste.

In individual serving bowls or a large serving dish, start by adding a portion of cooked brown rice to each bowl. Next, add a generous scoop of the black beans on top of the rice.

Follow this with a serving of corn kernels and diced avocados. Sprinkle the finely chopped red onion over the bowl. Garnish with a generous amount of freshly chopped cilantro.

Squeeze fresh lime juice over each bowl for a zesty flavor. You can adjust the amount of lime juice to your liking. Sprinkle a pinch of ground cumin over each bowl for a hint of warm, smoky flavor. Season the bowl with salt and pepper to taste.

Using a fork or spoon, gently mix all the ingredients in the bowl to combine the flavors. Ensure that the avocado is distributed evenly throughout the bowl.

SAUTEED GREENS WITH WHITE BEANS

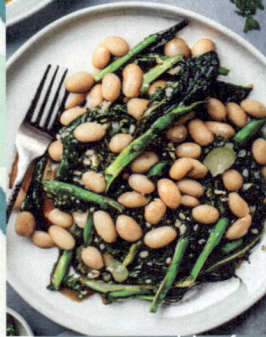

- Assorted leafy greens (kale, spinach, Swiss chard)
- 2 cans (15 oz each) white beans
- 2 cloves garlic
- Olive oil
- Fresh lemon juice
- Red pepper flakes (optional)
- Salt and pepper to taste

Wash and chop the assorted leafy greens of your choice (kale, spinach, Swiss chard, or a combination). You can use pre-washed and pre-chopped greens for convenience.

In a large skillet or frying pan, heat a few tablespoons of olive oil over medium heat.

Add the minced garlic to the hot olive oil. Sauté for about 30 seconds or until the garlic becomes fragrant but not browned.

Carefully add the chopped leafy greens to the skillet. Be cautious, as they may splatter initially due to moisture content.

Stir the greens gently to coat them evenly with the garlic-infused olive oil. Continue sautéing for about 3-5 minutes or until the greens start to wilt and become tender. They will reduce in volume as they cook.

Once the greens have wilted and become tender, add two cans of drained and rinsed white beans to the skillet.

Season the greens and beans with a generous squeeze of fresh lemon juice for a bright and zesty flavor. If you enjoy some heat, you can add a pinch of red pepper flakes at this point for a touch of spiciness. Season the mixture with salt and pepper to taste.

Continue sautéing the greens and white beans for an additional 2 minutes, allowing the flavors to meld and the beans to heat through.

Transfer the sautéed greens with white beans to a serving dish.

Delectable Main Courses for Health

BAKED HALIBUT WITH TOMATOES AND OLIVES

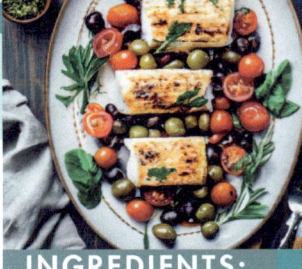

COOKING PROCESS:

Preheat your oven to 375°F (190°C). In a large ovenproof skillet or baking dish, heat the olive oil over medium heat.
Add the chopped onion and sauté for about 3-4 minutes, or until the onion becomes translucent and starts to soften. Stir in the minced garlic and sauté for an additional 30 seconds until fragrant. Add the diced tomatoes (with their juices) to the skillet. Stir in the sliced Kalamata olives, capers, and dried oregano. Season with salt and black pepper to taste.
Bring the tomato mixture to a simmer and cook for about 5-7 minutes, or until the sauce thickens slightly. While the tomato sauce is simmering, season the halibut fillets with a pinch of salt and black pepper. Nestle the halibut fillets into the tomato mixture in the skillet or baking dish.
Transfer the skillet or dish to the preheated oven and bake for approximately 15-20 minutes, or until the halibut is cooked through and flakes easily with a fork. The exact cooking time may vary based on the thickness of your halibut fillets, so keep an eye on them.
Once the halibut is done, remove the skillet or dish from the oven. Garnish with fresh basil leaves (if using) and serve hot. Serve with lemon wedges on the side for an extra burst of flavor.

INGREDIENTS:
- 4 halibut fillets (about 6 ounces each)
- 2 tbsp olive oil
- 1 onion
- 3 cloves garlic
- 1 can (14 ounces) diced tomatoes (or use fresh tomatoes)
- 1/2 cup Kalamata olives pitted
- 2 tbsp capers
- 1 tsp dried oregano
- Salt and black pepper
- Fresh basil leaves for garnish
- Lemon wedges for serving

BAKED SALMON WITH LEMON AND DILL

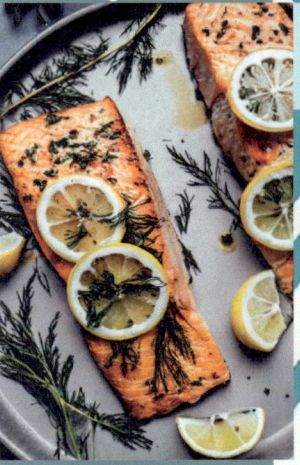

Preheat your oven to 375°F (190°C). Ensure it's fully preheated before you start cooking.
Place salmon fillets on a clean surface, such as a cutting board or a plate. Season both sides of each fillet with olive oil, minced garlic, chopped fresh dill, salt, and pepper. Press the seasonings gently onto the surface of the salmon to adhere.
Line a baking sheet or baking dish with aluminum foil or parchment paper to make cleanup easier. Place lemon slices on the lined sheet, creating a bed for the salmon fillets to sit on. The lemon slices will infuse the salmon with a fresh, citrusy flavor and prevent it from sticking to the foil.
Carefully place each seasoned salmon fillet on top of the lemon slices on the baking sheet. Ensure they are evenly spaced.
For an extra burst of flavor, you can add additional lemon slices on top of each salmon fillet. Sprinkle a bit more chopped dill on top of each fillet for added freshness.
Place the baking sheet with the salmon in the preheated oven. Bake for approximately 15-20 minutes, or until the salmon is cooked through and flakes easily with a fork. The exact cooking time may vary depending on the thickness of the fillets.
Once the salmon is done, remove it from the oven. Allow the salmon to rest for a few minutes. This helps the juices redistribute and keeps the fish moist.

- 4 salmon fillets
- Fresh dill
- Lemon slices
- 2 cloves garlic
- Olive oil
- Salt and pepper to taste

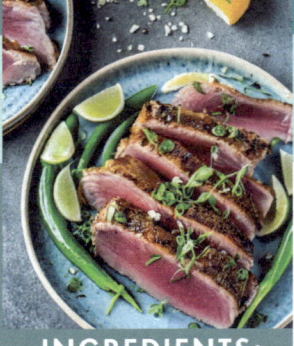

OKINAWAN SEARED TUNA STEAK

INGREDIENTS:

- 4 tuna steaks (about 6 ounces each)
- 2 tablespoons soy sauce
- 1 tablespoon rice vinegar
- 1 tablespoon mirin (sweet rice wine)
- 2 cloves garlic
- 1 teaspoon grated fresh ginger
- 2 tablespoons sesame seeds
- 1 tablespoon vegetable oil
- Salt and black pepper, to taste
- Sliced green onions
- Lemon wedges

COOKING PROCESS:

In a mixing bowl, whisk together the soy sauce, rice vinegar, mirin, minced garlic, and grated ginger to create the marinade.

Place the tuna steaks in a shallow dish or a resealable plastic bag and pour the marinade over them. Ensure that the tuna is coated evenly. Marinate for at least 30 minutes, or refrigerate for up to 2 hours for more flavor.

While the tuna is marinating, spread the sesame seeds on a plate. After marinating, remove the tuna steaks from the marinade, allowing any excess liquid to drip off.

Season both sides of the tuna steaks with a pinch of salt and black pepper.

Press each side of the tuna steaks into the sesame seeds to coat them generously.

Heat the vegetable oil in a skillet or frying pan over high heat.

Once the oil is hot, carefully add the tuna steaks. Sear the tuna for about 1-2 minutes per side for rare or longer if you prefer it more well-done. Keep in mind that tuna cooks quickly, so be attentive to prevent overcooking.

Transfer the seared tuna steaks to a cutting board and let them rest for a minute or two.

Slice the tuna steaks into thin, even slices.

Garnish with sliced green onions (if using) and serve with lemon wedges on the side.

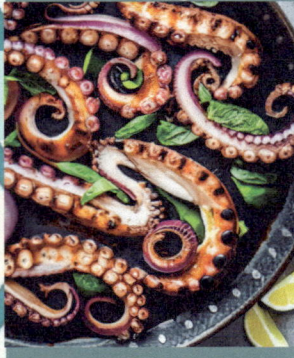

GRILLED OCTOPUS

- 2 pounds octopus
- 2-3 large lemons
- 4 cloves garlic
- 1/4 cup extra-virgin olive oil
- 2 teaspoons dried oregano
- Salt and black pepper, to taste
- Lemon wedges and fresh parsley for garnish (optional)

Start by cleaning the octopus. Rinse it thoroughly under cold running water and remove any remaining beak or skin. You can choose to either cook the octopus whole or separate the tentacles. If using whole, make sure to score the body of the octopus with a sharp knife to allow for even cooking and better flavor absorption.

In a large bowl, combine the lemon juice, minced garlic, extra-virgin olive oil, dried oregano, salt, and black pepper. This will be your marinade.

Place the cleaned octopus in the marinade, ensuring it's well-coated. Cover the bowl and refrigerate for at least 2 hours or overnight for best results.

Preheat your grill to medium-high heat (about 400-450°F or 200-230°C). Make sure to clean and oil the grill grates to prevent sticking.

Remove the marinated octopus from the bowl and let any excess marinade drip off.

Place the octopus on the grill, tentacles down, and cook for about 2-3 minutes per side. The tentacles should become slightly charred and curl up. Be mindful not to overcook, as octopus can become tough. It's best when it's tender and slightly charred on the outside.

VIBRANT SUSHI BOWLS

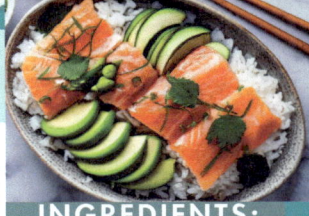

COOKING PROCESS:

Rinse the sushi rice in a fine-mesh strainer until the water runs clear. In a saucepan, combine the rinsed rice and water. Bring to a boil over high heat, then reduce the heat to low, cover, and simmer for 15 minutes. Remove from heat and let it sit, covered, for an additional 10 minutes.
In a small saucepan, heat the rice vinegar, sugar, and salt over low heat until the sugar and salt dissolve. Once the rice is cooked, transfer it to a large bowl, and while it's still hot, drizzle the seasoned vinegar over it. Gently fold the rice with a wooden or plastic spatula to combine. Allow the rice to cool to room temperature.
While the rice is cooling, prepare the toppings. Slice the sushi-grade raw salmon or tuna into thin strips. Thinly slice the cucumber and avocado. Shred the nori into small pieces using scissors.
Divide the seasoned sushi rice equally among four bowls. Arrange the sliced fish, cucumber, and avocado on top of the rice in each bowl. Sprinkle shredded nori over the toppings.
Place small bowls of pickled ginger, soy sauce, and wasabi paste on the side for diners to add as they like. You can also sprinkle sesame seeds and sliced green onions for extra flavor and garnish.

INGREDIENTS:
For the Rice:
- 2 cups sushi rice
- 2 cups water
- 1/4 cup rice vinegar
- 2 tbsp sugar
- 1 tsp salt

For the Toppings:
- 8 ounces sushi-grade raw salmon or tuna
- 1 cucumber
- 1 avocado
- 1 cup shredded nori (dried seaweed sheets)
- 1/2 cup pickled ginger
- 1/4 cup soy sauce
- 1/4 cup wasabi paste
- 1 tbsp sesame seeds (optional)
- Green onions

SARDINIAN FREGOLA WITH CLAMS

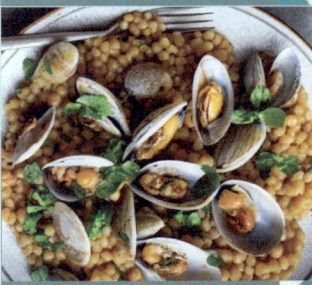

Bring a large pot of salted water to a boil. Add the fregola pasta and cook according to the package instructions until al dente. Drain and set aside.
In a large skillet or pan, heat the olive oil over medium heat. Add the finely chopped onion and sauté for about 2-3 minutes until it becomes translucent. Add the minced garlic and dried red pepper flakes to the skillet. Sauté for another 30 seconds until fragrant.
Pour in the dry white wine and allow it to simmer for about 2-3 minutes to cook off the alcohol.
Stir in the diced tomatoes and their juices. Simmer for about 5-7 minutes, allowing the sauce to thicken slightly. Gently add the cleaned clams to the skillet. Cover the pan and let them steam for about 5-7 minutes. The clams are done when they open. Discard any that do not open.
Carefully remove the opened clams from the skillet and set them aside. Add the cooked fregola pasta to the tomato and clam broth in the skillet. Stir to combine and let it simmer for another 2-3 minutes to heat through.
Season the fregola and clam mixture with salt and black pepper to taste. If you like it spicy, you can add more red pepper flakes at this stage. Return the cooked clams to the skillet and gently mix.
Transfer the Sardinian Fregola with Clams to serving plates or a large platter. Garnish with chopped fresh parsley and serve with lemon wedges on the side for squeezing over the dish.

- 1 1/2 cups fregola pasta
- 1 pound fresh clams
- 2 tablespoons olive oil
- 1 small onion
- 2 cloves garlic
- 1/2 cup dry white wine
- 1 can (14 ounces) diced tomatoes
- 1 teaspoon dried red pepper flakes (adjust to taste)
- Salt and black pepper to taste
- Fresh parsley
- Lemon wedges

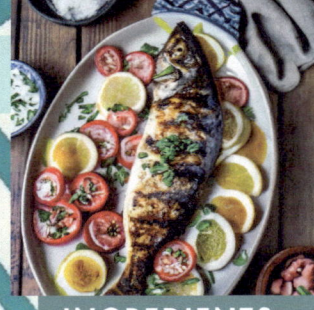

GRILLED WHOLE SEA BASS

INGREDIENTS:

- 2 whole sea bass, cleaned and gutted (about 1.5 to 2 pounds each)
- 2 lemons
- 4-6 cloves garlic
- 1/4 cup fresh parsley 1/4 cup fresh dill
- 1/4 cup olive oil
- Salt and freshly ground black pepper, to taste
- Lemon wedges

COOKING PROCESS:

Preheat your grill to medium-high heat, around 350-400°F (175-200°C). Make sure to clean and oil the grill grates to prevent sticking. Prepare the sea bass by rinsing them inside and out under cold running water. Pat them dry with paper towels.

In a small bowl, combine the minced garlic, chopped parsley, chopped dill, and extra-virgin olive oil. This mixture will serve as a flavorful marinade for the fish.

Season the sea bass generously, both inside and outside, with salt and freshly ground black pepper. Stuff the cavity of each sea bass with lemon slices. This will infuse the fish with a bright, citrusy flavor. Brush the fish all over with the herb and olive oil mixture. Make sure to coat them evenly.

Once the grill is hot and ready, place the sea bass directly on the grates. Grill them for about 5-7 minutes per side, or until the flesh flakes easily with a fork and the skin is nicely charred. The exact cooking time may vary depending on the thickness of the fish, so keep an eye on them.

Carefully flip the sea bass using a large spatula or grill tongs to grill the other side.

While the fish is grilling, you can continue to brush them with the herb and olive oil mixture for added flavor.

Once the sea bass is fully cooked, remove them from the grill and transfer them to a serving platter. Garnish with additional fresh herbs and lemon wedges.

EASY TERIYAKI SALMON

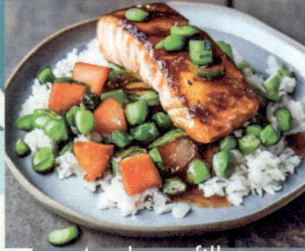

- 4 salmon fillets (about 6-8 ounces each)
- 1/2 cup low-sodium soy sauce
- 1/4 cup mirin (sweet rice wine)
- 1/4 cup sake (Japanese rice wine) or dry white wine
- 2 tablespoons sugar (white or brown)
- 2 cloves garlic
- 1-inch piece of fresh ginger
- 2 tablespoons vegetable oil (for cooking)
- Optional garnishes: sesame seeds, green onions

In a small saucepan, combine the soy sauce, mirin, sake (or white wine), sugar, minced garlic, and grated ginger. Stir well.

Place the saucepan over medium heat and bring the mixture to a simmer. Reduce the heat to low and simmer gently for about 10-15 minutes, or until the sauce thickens slightly. Stir occasionally to prevent burning.

While the teriyaki sauce is simmering, heat a large skillet or frying pan over medium-high heat. Add the vegetable oil and allow it to get hot.

Season the salmon fillets with a pinch of salt and freshly ground black pepper. Carefully add the salmon fillets to the hot skillet, skin-side down if using skin-on fillets. Cook for about 2-3 minutes on each side, or until the salmon is nicely seared and has a golden-brown color. If your fillets have skin, the skin should become crispy.

Once the salmon is seared on both sides, pour the teriyaki sauce over the fillets in the skillet. Reduce the heat to medium-low and simmer the salmon in the teriyaki sauce for an additional 2-3 minutes, or until the salmon is cooked to your desired level of doneness. Baste the salmon with the sauce as it cooks.

Remove the skillet from the heat and transfer the teriyaki salmon fillets to a serving platter. Spoon some of the teriyaki sauce over the salmon and garnish with sesame seeds and sliced green onions, if desired.

Seafood Specials for Wellness

EXOTIC MISO-GLAZED SALMON

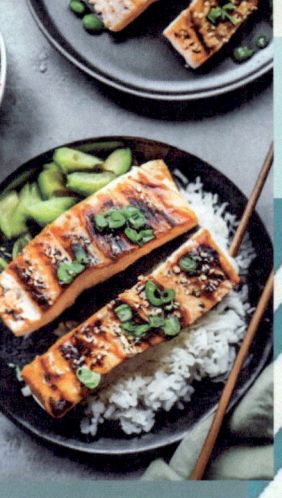

COOKING PROCESS:

In a small saucepan, combine the white miso paste, mirin, sake, sugar, and soy sauce. Heat the mixture over low heat, stirring constantly, until the sugar has completely dissolved, and the mixture has become smooth and well-blended. This step is important as it helps to infuse the flavors of the ingredients together. Once done, remove the saucepan from the heat source and allow the mixture to cool down naturally to reach room temperature.

Next, prepare the salmon fillets in a shallow dish or a resealable plastic bag. Pour half of the cooled miso glaze over the salmon, ensuring each fillet is generously coated with the flavorful mixture. The remaining glaze should be reserved for later use. To enhance the taste, it is recommended to let the salmon marinate in the glaze for at least 30 minutes in the refrigerator. However, if you have more time, marinating it for a few hours or even overnight will result in a deeper and more pronounced flavor profile.

Meanwhile, preheat your oven to 400°F (200°C) to ensure that it reaches the optimal temperature for cooking the salmon to perfection. While the oven is heating up, heat a large oven-safe skillet over medium-high heat. Add the vegetable oil to the hot skillet and allow it to heat up until it starts to shimmer, indicating that it is ready for the salmon. Carefully remove the salmon fillets from the marinade, allowing any excess glaze to drip off, and place them in the skillet, ensuring that the skin side is facing down. This will help in achieving crispy and delicious skin.

Sear the salmon fillets in the skillet for approximately 2-3 minutes, or until the skin turns crispy and golden brown. This initial step of searing helps to lock in the flavors and create a delightful texture. To further enhance the taste, brush the tops of the salmon fillets with some reserved miso glaze, adding an extra layer of sweetness and umami goodness.

Now it's time to transfer the skillet to the preheated oven, where the salmon will continue to cook and become tender and juicy. Bake the salmon for approximately 8-10 minutes, or until it is fully cooked through and easily flakes apart when tested with a fork. Remember that the cooking time may vary depending on the thickness of your salmon fillets, so it's always good to keep an eye on them to ensure they are cooked to your desired level of doneness.

Once the salmon is done, remove it from the oven and let it rest for a few minutes before serving. This resting period allows the juices to redistribute within the fish, resulting in a moist and flavorful final dish. You can serve the miso-glazed salmon as is or pair it with your favorite side dishes for a complete and satisfying meal.

INGREDIENTS:

- 4 salmon fillets (about 6 ounces each)
- 1/4 cup white miso paste
- 2 tablespoons mirin (Japanese sweet rice wine)
- 2 tablespoons sake (Japanese rice wine)
- 2 tablespoons sugar
- 2 tablespoons soy sauce
- 1 tablespoon vegetable oil
- Sesame seeds and sliced green onions for garnish (optional)

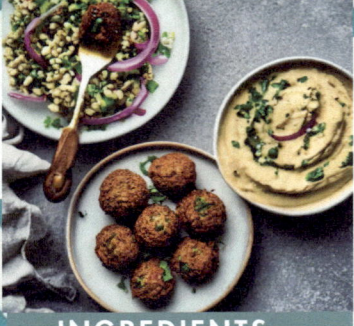

FALAFEL WITH HUMMUS AND BULGUR SALAD

INGREDIENTS:

For the Falafel:
- 2 cups canned chickpeas
- 1 small onion
- 2 cloves garlic
- 1 tsp ground cumin
- 1 tsp ground coriander
- 1/4 tsp cayenne pepper (adjust to taste)
- 1 cup fresh parsley
- 1/2 cup fresh cilantro
- 1 tsp baking powder
- Salt and black pepper to taste
- Vegetable oil for frying

For the Hummus:
- 1 can (15 ounces) chickpeas
- 1/4 cup fresh lemon juice (about 1 large lemon)
- 1/4 cup well-stirred tahini
- 1 small garlic clove
- 2 tbsp extra-virgin olive oil, plus more for serving
- 1/2 tsp ground cumin
- Salt to taste
- 2 to 3 tbsp water, as needed
- Paprika and fresh parsley for garnish

For the Bulgur Salad:
- 1 cup bulgur wheat
- 1 1/2 cups boiling water
- 1 1/2 cups fresh parsley
- 1/2 cup fresh mint leaves
- 3 tomatoes
- 1 cucumber
- 1/2 red onion
- 1/4 cup extra-virgin olive oil
- Juice of 2 lemons
- Salt and black pepper

COOKING PROCESS:

For the Falafel:
Prepare the chickpeas by draining and rinsing them with water. In a food processor, combine the drained chickpeas, chopped onion, minced garlic, ground cumin, ground coriander, cayenne pepper, fresh parsley, fresh cilantro, baking powder, salt, and black pepper.
Pulse the mixture in the food processor until well combined but not a smooth paste. You should still have some texture.
Using your hands, shape the mixture into small patties or balls (about 1.5 inches in diameter). Place them on a baking sheet lined with parchment paper.
In a deep skillet or frying pan, heat vegetable oil over medium-high heat until it reaches about 350°F (180°C).
Carefully place the falafel patties or balls into the hot oil and fry for about 3-4 minutes on each side or until they are golden brown and crispy. Remove with a slotted spoon and place them on a plate lined with paper towels to drain any excess oil.

For the Hummus:
Prepare the chickpeas by draining and rinsing them with water. In a food processor, combine the chickpeas, lemon juice, tahini, minced garlic, olive oil, ground cumin, and a pinch of salt.
Blend until smooth. If the mixture is too thick, you can add 2 to 3 tablespoons of water to achieve your desired consistency.
Taste the hummus and adjust the salt and lemon juice if needed. You can also drizzle a bit of extra-virgin olive oil on top and garnish with paprika and chopped fresh parsley.

For the Bulgur Salad:
Place the bulgur wheat in a bowl and pour boiling water over it. Cover and let it sit for about 20 minutes, or until the bulgur is tender and has absorbed the water.
Fluff the bulgur with a fork and allow it to cool to room temperature.
In a large mixing bowl, combine the cooled bulgur, chopped parsley, chopped mint, diced tomatoes, diced cucumber, chopped red onion, extra-virgin olive oil, lemon juice, salt, and black pepper. Toss everything together until well mixed. Arrange the Falafel on a plate, accompanied by a bowl of Hummus and a serving of Bulgur Salad. You can also serve them in pita bread or flatbread as sandwiches or wraps.

MEDITERRANEAN STUFFED GRAPE LEAVES

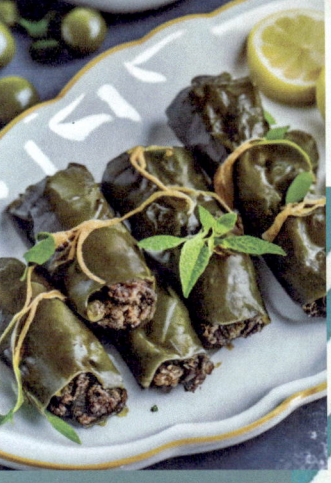

COOKING PROCESS:

Remove the grape leaves from the jar and rinse them thoroughly under cold running water to remove excess brine. Drain them and set aside.

Prepare the Filling (Optional): In a skillet, brown the ground beef or lamb over medium-high heat until it's fully cooked. If you're not using meat, skip this step.

Add the finely chopped onion and minced garlic to the skillet with the cooked meat (or directly to the next step if not using meat).

Sauté the onion and garlic until they become translucent.

In a mixing bowl, combine the long-grain white rice, fresh lemon juice, extra virgin olive oil, chopped fresh dill, chopped fresh mint, and optional toasted pine nuts and currants or raisins (if using).

If you've browned meat and sautéed onion and garlic in step 2, add them to the mixing bowl as well.

Season the rice mixture with salt and pepper to taste. Start with a pinch of each and adjust based on your preference.

Place one grape leaf on a clean work surface with the shiny side down and the stem end facing you.

Place about a teaspoon of the rice filling (or meat and rice filling) in the center of the leaf, near the stem end. Fold the sides of the leaf over the filling, then roll it up tightly, similar to rolling a burrito.

Repeat this process for the remaining grape leaves and filling.

In a large pot, arrange the stuffed grape leaves in a single layer. Pour enough water into the pot to just cover the stuffed grape leaves.

Place a heatproof plate or an overturned ovenproof dish on top of the grape leaves to keep them submerged during cooking.

Cover the pot and bring it to a boil. Then, reduce the heat and simmer for approximately 45-60 minutes, or until the rice is fully cooked and the grape leaves are tender.

Check the water level periodically and add more if necessary to prevent the grape leaves from drying out.

Once cooked, remove the Mediterranean Stuffed Grape Leaves from the pot and transfer them to a serving platter.

INGREDIENTS:

For the Grape Leaves:

- 1 jar of grape leaves in brine (approximately 60-80 grape leaves)
- 1 cup long-grain white rice (jasmine or basmati)
- 1/2 cup fresh lemon juice
- 1/4 cup extra virgin olive oil
- 1/4 cup fresh dill
- 1/4 cup fresh mint
- 1 small onion
- 2 cloves garlic
- Salt and pepper

For the Filling:

- 1/2 pound ground beef or lamb (optional)
- 1/2 cup pine nuts, toasted (optional)
- 1/4 cup currants or raisins (optional)

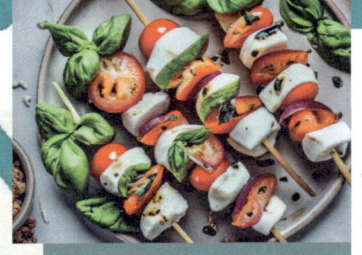

CAPRESE SKEWERS

INGREDIENTS:

- 16 fresh cherry tomatoes
- 16 fresh small mozzarella ball (bocconcini or ciliegine)
- Fresh basil leaves
- Extra virgin olive oil
- Balsamic glaze (optional)
- Wooden skewers (4-6 inches in length)
- Salt and pepper to taste

COOKING PROCESS:

Wash and dry the cherry tomatoes.
Drain the mozzarella balls if they are stored in liquid. Wash and pat dry the fresh basil leaves. Soak the wooden skewers in water for about 15-20 minutes to prevent them from splintering or burning when you assemble the skewers.
Take a wooden skewer and start by threading a cherry tomato onto it. Follow the tomato with a small mozzarella ball. Next, add a fresh basil leaf. Repeat this process until you have four cherry tomatoes, four mozzarella balls, and four basil leaves on each skewer. Continue assembling the remaining skewers.
Arrange the Caprese skewers on a serving platter. Drizzle extra virgin olive oil over the skewers. Season with a pinch of salt and pepper to taste.
If you like, you can drizzle a balsamic glaze over the skewers for extra flavor and presentation. This step is optional but adds a sweet and tangy dimension to the dish.

OKINAWAN BRAISED PORK BELLY

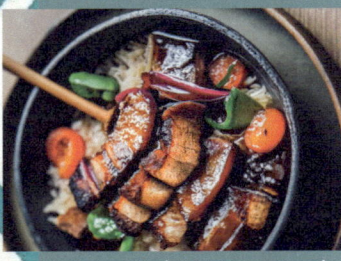

- 1 pound (450 g) pork belly, skin-on
- 1 tablespoon vegetable oil
- 1 large onion
- 2 cloves garlic
- 1 thumb-sized piece of ginger
- 2 cups (480 ml) water
- 1/2 cup (120 ml) soy sauce
- 1/4 cup (60 ml) mirin (Japanese rice wine)
- 1/4 cup (60 ml) sake (Japanese rice wine)
- 1/4 cup (60 g) brown sugar
- 2 star anise pods
- 2-3 dried shiitake mushrooms
- 1-2 carrots (optional)
- Steamed white rice, for serving
- Green onions, for garnish (optional)

Start by preparing the pork belly. If it's not already sliced, cut it into bite-sized pieces, ensuring the skin is included. Rinse and pat dry with paper towels.
Heat a large, heavy-bottomed pot or Dutch oven over medium-high heat. Add the vegetable oil and let it heat up.
Carefully place the pork belly pieces, skin side down, in the hot oil. Allow them to sear and develop a golden-brown crust on all sides. This may take about 5-7 minutes. Remove the pork from the pot and set it aside.
In the same pot, add the minced garlic and ginger. Sauté them for about a minute until fragrant. Add the thinly sliced onion and cook until it becomes translucent, which will take about 5 minutes. Return the seared pork belly to the pot, and add the carrots if you're using them. Pour in the soy sauce, mirin, sake, and water. Add the brown sugar, star anise pods, and dried shiitake mushrooms. Stir to combine.
Bring the mixture to a boil, then reduce the heat to low.
Cover the pot and simmer for about 1.5 to 2 hours, or until the pork belly becomes tender and the flavors meld together. Stir occasionally to prevent sticking. While the pork is simmering, prepare steamed white rice according to your preference.
Once the pork is tender, remove the star anise pods and shiitake mushrooms from the pot. Serve the Okinawan Braised Pork Belly over steamed white rice. Garnish with thinly sliced green onions if desired.

Global Flavors and Longevity

SARDINIAN LAMB AND ARTICHOKE STEW

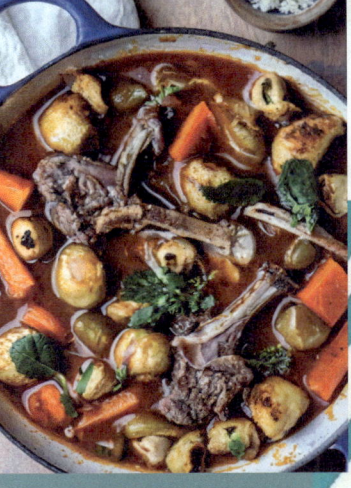

COOKING PROCESS:

Begin by preparing the fresh artichokes if using. Trim the tough outer leaves, cut off the top third of each artichoke, and trim the stem.
Quarter them and remove the fuzzy choke from the center.
Place the prepared artichoke quarters in a bowl of water with lemon juice to prevent browning.
Heat the extra-virgin olive oil in a large, heavy-bottomed pot or Dutch oven over medium-high heat.
Add the chopped onion and minced garlic.
Sauté for about 2-3 minutes until the onion becomes translucent and fragrant.
Add the bite-sized pieces of lamb to the pot.
Sear them on all sides until they develop a golden-brown crust.
This may take about 5-7 minutes.
Pour in the dry white wine and allow it to simmer for a few minutes, scraping up any flavorful bits from the bottom of the pot.
Add the diced tomatoes, dried oregano, dried thyme, salt, and black pepper to the pot.
Stir everything together.
Drain the prepared artichoke quarters and add them to the pot.
Reduce the heat to low, cover the pot, and let the stew simmer gently for about 1.5 to 2 hours.
This allows the lamb to become tender and the flavors to meld together.
Stir occasionally.
Taste and adjust the seasoning with more salt and pepper if needed.
Once the lamb is tender and the artichokes are cooked through, your Sardinian Lamb and Artichoke Stew is ready to serve.
Garnish the stew with freshly chopped parsley and serve it hot.
You can also offer lemon wedges on the side for a touch of brightness if desired.

INGREDIENTS:

- 1.5 pounds (680 g) boneless lamb shoulder, cut into bite-sized pieces
- 4-6 fresh artichokes (or 1 can of artichoke hearts, drained and quartered)
- 2 tablespoons extra-virgin olive oil
- 1 onion
- 2 cloves garlic
- 1 cup (240 ml) dry white wine
- 1 can (14 ounces/400 g) diced tomatoes
- 1 teaspoon dried oregano
- 1 teaspoon dried thyme
- Salt and black pepper, to taste
- Fresh parsley, for garnish
- Lemon wedges, for serving (optional)

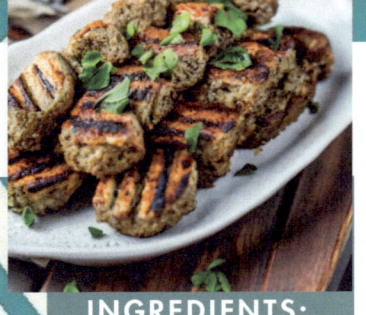

BIFTEKIA (GRILLED MEAT PATTIES)

INGREDIENTS:
- 1 pound (450 g) ground lean beef or a combination of beef and lamb
- 1 small onion
- 2 cloves garlic
- 1/4 cup fresh breadcrumbs
- 1/4 cup fresh parsley
- 1/4 cup fresh mint
- 1/2 tsp dried oregano
- Salt and black pepper, to taste
- 1 egg
- Olive oil, for brushing

COOKING PROCESS:

Start by preheating your grill or barbecue to medium-high heat. In a mixing bowl, combine the ground meat (beef or a combination of beef and lamb) with the finely grated onion, minced garlic, fresh breadcrumbs, chopped parsley, chopped mint, dried oregano, salt, and black pepper. Use your hands to mix the ingredients thoroughly.

Crack the egg into the mixture and continue to mix until everything is well combined. The egg helps bind the mixture together. With clean hands, shape the mixture into oval or round patties, each about the size of your palm and about 1/2 inch thick. You should be able to make around 4 patties from this mixture. Place the meat patties on a tray or plate and brush them lightly with olive oil. This will help prevent sticking to the grill.

Once the grill is hot, place the meat patties on the grill grates. Grill them for about 3-4 minutes on each side, or until they develop a nice char and are cooked to your desired level of doneness. You can cook them longer for well-done or shorter for medium-rare. While grilling, avoid pressing down on the patties with a spatula as this can release juices and make them dry.

Once the biftekia are cooked to your liking, remove them from the grill and allow them to rest for a few minutes.

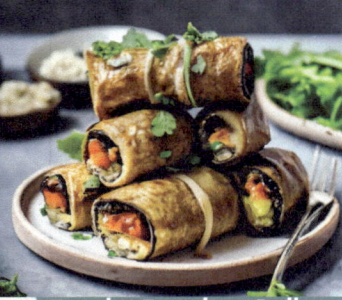

EGGPLANT AND WALNUT ROLLS

For the Eggplant Rolls:
- 2 large eggplants
- Salt
- Vegetable oil

For the Walnut Sauce:
- 1 cup walnuts, shelled
- 2-3 cloves garlic
- 1 tsp ground coriander
- 1 tsp ground fenugreek (optional)
- 1/2 tsp cayenne pepper or paprika
- 1 tbsp wine vinegar white or red
- Salt to taste
- Fresh cilantro or parsley leaves

Slice the eggplants lengthwise into thin strips (about 1/4-inch thick). Sprinkle salt over the eggplant slices and let them sit for about 15-20 minutes. This helps remove excess moisture and bitterness. After the resting period, rinse the eggplant slices under cold water and pat them dry with paper towels.

Heat vegetable oil in a large skillet over medium-high heat. Once the oil is hot, add the eggplant slices in batches and fry until they are soft and lightly browned on both sides.

Place them on paper towels to drain excess oil.

In a mixing bowl, combine the finely ground walnuts, minced garlic, ground coriander, ground fenugreek (if using), and cayenne pepper or paprika. Add the vinegar and mix well. The mixture will become thick.

Take a fried eggplant slice and place a small amount of the walnut sauce at one end. Roll the eggplant slice, enclosing the sauce, to form a roll or cylinder. Repeat with the remaining eggplant slices and walnut sauce.

Arrange the eggplant rolls on a serving platter. Garnish with fresh cilantro or parsley leaves.

SPANAKOPITA (SPINACH PIE)

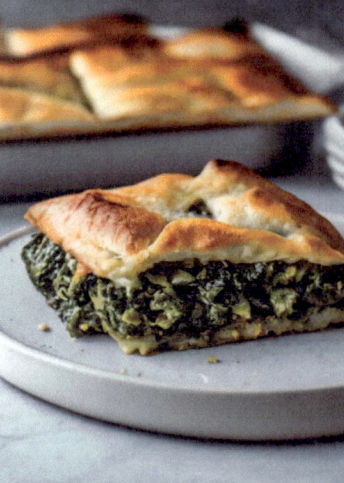

COOKING PROCESS:

For the Filling:

In a large skillet, heat 2 tablespoons of olive oil over medium heat. Add the finely chopped onion and minced garlic. Sauté until the onions become translucent, about 2-3 minutes.
Add the chopped spinach to the skillet. Cook and stir until the spinach wilts and any excess liquid evaporates, about 5-7 minutes. Remove from heat and allow it to cool slightly.
In a large mixing bowl, combine the cooked spinach mixture, crumbled feta cheese, chopped fresh dill, chopped fresh parsley, salt, black pepper, and a pinch of ground nutmeg (if using). Mix well to create the filling. Taste and adjust seasoning as needed.

For Assembly:

Preheat your oven to 350°F (175°C). Carefully unroll the thawed phyllo dough sheets and cover them with a clean kitchen towel to keep them from drying out as you work.
Take one sheet of phyllo dough and brush it lightly with melted butter. Place another sheet on top and brush it with more melted butter. Repeat this process until you have a stack of 8 sheets.
Spread half of the spinach and feta filling evenly over the phyllo stack.
Continue layering and brushing phyllo sheets on top of the filling until you have used all 16 sheets, brushing each sheet with melted butter as you go.
Spread the remaining spinach and feta filling evenly on top of the last phyllo sheet. Carefully fold in the excess phyllo dough from the sides over the filling, and then roll the phyllo stack from the bottom to the top to create a log. Place the seam side down.
Brush the top of the spanakopita with more melted butter and olive oil. Use a sharp knife to score the top of the spanakopita diagonally into diamond or square-shaped portions.
Place the spanakopita in the preheated oven and bake for 40-45 minutes or until it is golden brown and crispy. Remove from the oven and let it cool for a few minutes before slicing along the scored lines. Sprinkle sesame seeds on top if desired.

INGREDIENTS:

For the Filling:
- 1 pound fresh spinach
- 1 cup feta cheese
- 1 small onion
- 2 cloves garlic
- 2 tablespoons olive oil
- 1/4 cup fresh dill (or 2 teaspoons dried dill)
- 1/4 cup fresh parsley
- Salt and black pepper to taste
- Pinch of ground nutmeg (optional)

For the Phyllo Dough and Assembly:
- 1 package of frozen phyllo dough (16 sheets)
- 1/2 cup unsalted butter
- Olive oil for brushing
- Sesame seeds for garnish (optional)

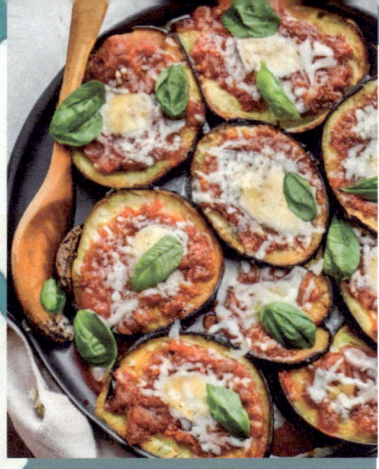

MEDITERRANEAN BAKED EGGPLANT PARMESAN

INGREDIENTS:

For the Eggplant:
- 2 large eggplants
- Salt
- Olive oil

For the Tomato Sauce:
- 2 tablespoons olive oil
- 1 onion
- 2 cloves garlic
- 1 can (28 ounces) crushed tomatoes
- 1 teaspoon dried basil
- 1 teaspoon dried oregano
- Salt and black pepper to taste
- Fresh basil leaves, for garnish (optional)

For the Cheese Mixture:
- 1 1/2 cups ricotta cheese
- 1/2 cup grated Parmesan cheese
- 1/2 cup shredded mozzarella cheese
- 1 egg
- Salt and black pepper to taste

For Assembly:
- 1 cup shredded mozzarella cheese
- Fresh basil leaves, for garnish (optional)

COOKING PROCESS:

To begin, peel the eggplant and slice it into 1/2-inch thick rounds. Place the eggplant slices in a single layer on a baking sheet. Sprinkle each slice lightly with salt and let them sit for about 30 minutes. This helps to remove excess moisture and bitterness from the eggplant. After 30 minutes, pat the eggplant slices dry with paper towels.

Preheat your oven to 375°F (190°C).

Brush both sides of the eggplant slices with olive oil. Arrange them in a single layer on baking sheets. Roast in the preheated oven for about 15-20 minutes or until they are tender and slightly golden. Remove from the oven and set aside.

In a large saucepan, heat 2 tablespoons of olive oil over medium heat. Add the finely chopped onion and minced garlic. Sauté for about 5 minutes until they become translucent and fragrant. Stir in the crushed tomatoes, dried basil, dried oregano, salt, and black pepper. Simmer for about 15-20 minutes, stirring occasionally, until the sauce thickens.

In a bowl, combine the ricotta cheese, grated Parmesan cheese, shredded mozzarella cheese, one egg, salt, and black pepper. Mix until well combined.

In a baking dish, spread a thin layer of tomato sauce on the bottom. Place a layer of roasted eggplant slices on top of the sauce. Spoon some of the cheese mixture over the eggplant. Repeat with another layer of eggplant, tomato sauce, and cheese mixture until you've used all your ingredients, finishing with a layer of tomato sauce on top.

Sprinkle the top with 1 cup of shredded mozzarella cheese. Cover the baking dish with aluminum foil and bake in the preheated oven for 25-30 minutes. Then, remove the foil and bake for an additional 10-15 minutes, or until the cheese is bubbly and golden brown.

Remove the Mediterranean Baked Eggplant Parmesan from the oven and let it cool for a few minutes.

Garnish with fresh basil leaves if desired. Slice and serve warm.

EGGPLANT AND ZUCCHINI RATATOUILLE

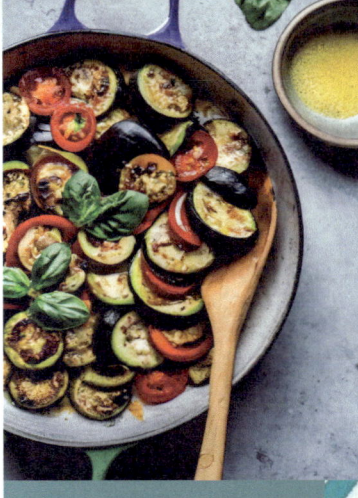

COOKING PROCESS:

Start by peeling the eggplant and zucchini, then proceed to dice them into 1-inch cubes.
Place the diced eggplant in a large colander, sprinkle with salt, and let it sit for about 30 minutes. This helps remove excess moisture and bitterness from the eggplant.
After 30 minutes, rinse the eggplant thoroughly and pat it dry with paper towels.
In a large skillet or a Dutch oven, heat the olive oil over medium heat.
Add the chopped onion and minced garlic, and sauté for about 2-3 minutes until they become fragrant and translucent.
Add the diced red and yellow bell peppers to the skillet and sauté for another 3-4 minutes until they begin to soften.
Stir in the crushed tomatoes, diced tomatoes, and tomato paste.
Mix well.
Add the dried basil, dried oregano, salt, and black pepper to the skillet.
Stir to combine. Reduce the heat to low, cover, and simmer for about 15-20 minutes, allowing the flavors to meld and the sauce to thicken.
While the sauce is simmering, in a separate skillet, heat a bit of olive oil over medium-high heat.
Add the diced eggplant and zucchini cubes.
Sauté for about 5-7 minutes, or until they become tender and slightly golden. Remove from heat.
Add the sautéed eggplant and zucchini to the tomato sauce.
Stir gently to combine all the ingredients.
Let it simmer for an additional 5 minutes to ensure the vegetables are fully cooked.
Taste and adjust the seasoning as needed.
You can add more salt, pepper, or dried herbs if desired.
Garnish with fresh basil leaves, if available.
Italian Eggplant and Zucchini Ratatouille can be served hot as a main dish or a side dish.
It pairs well with crusty bread, pasta, or rice.

INGREDIENTS:

- 1 large eggplant
- 2 zucchini
- 1 onion
- 2 cloves garlic
- 1 red bell pepper
- 1 yellow bell pepper
- 1 can (14 ounces) crushed tomatoes
- 1 can (14 ounces) diced tomatoes
- 2 tablespoons tomato paste
- 1 teaspoon dried basil
- 1 teaspoon dried oregano
- Salt and black pepper to taste
- 2 tablespoons olive oil
- Fresh basil leaves, for garnish (optional)

BAKED APPLES WITH CINNAMON

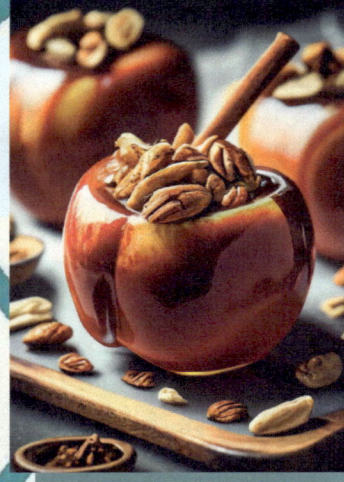

INGREDIENTS:

- 4 apples (e.g., Granny Smith, Honeycrisp, or your favorite variety)
- 2 tablespoons honey or maple syrup (adjust to taste)
- 1 teaspoon ground cinnamon
- 1/4 cup chopped nuts (e.g., walnuts, pecans, or almonds) - optional
- A pinch of salt (optional)
- 1/4 cup water or apple juice

COOKING PROCESS:

Preheat your oven to 375°F (190°C).
Wash and core the apples.
You can use an apple core or a small knife to remove the cores, leaving a well in the center for the filling.
In a small bowl, combine 2 tablespoons of honey or maple syrup (adjust to your desired sweetness) and 1 teaspoon of ground cinnamon.
If you like, you can also add a pinch of salt to enhance the flavors.
If you wish to include nuts, chopped 1/4 cup of your preferred nuts (e.g., walnuts, pecans, or almonds) and set them aside.
Place the cored apples in a baking dish.
Drizzle the honey-cinnamon mixture evenly over the apples, making sure to coat them inside the wells and around the exteriors.
If you're using nuts, stuff each apple well with a portion of the chopped nuts.
Pour 1/4 cup of water or apple juice into the bottom of the baking dish.
This will help keep the apples moist during baking.
Cover the baking dish with foil.
Bake the apples in the preheated oven for approximately 25-30 minutes, or until they become tender.
The exact baking time may vary depending on the size and type of apples, so check for doneness by inserting a fork into an apple to ensure it's soft and easily pierced.
Once the apples are tender, remove the foil and bake for an additional 5-10 minutes to allow the tops to caramelize and become slightly golden.
Carefully remove the baked apples from the oven and let them cool slightly before serving.
Serve the Baked Apples with Cinnamon as a warm and comforting dessert.
Optionally, you can drizzle any remaining juices from the baking dish over the apples for added flavor.

FIG AND WALNUT BARS

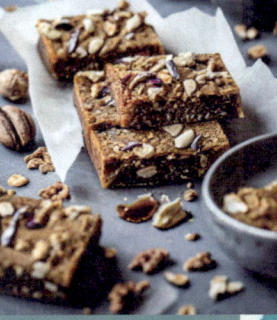

COOKING PROCESS:

Begin by preparing a square baking dish (about 8x8 inches) by lining it with parchment paper, leaving some overhang on the sides. This will make it easier to remove the bars later.

In a food processor, add: dried figs (stems removed), honey or maple syrup, creamy almond or peanut butter, vanilla extract, and a pinch of salt (if desired). Pulse the ingredients in the food processor until they form a sticky and cohesive mixture. This may take a minute or two. You want the figs to be well blended.

In a separate bowl, combine chopped walnuts, and old-fashioned oats. Pour the fig mixture from the food processor over the nuts and oats. Mix everything together until the ingredients are evenly distributed and form a thick, sticky mixture.

Transfer the mixture to the prepared baking dish. Use a spatula or your hands to press the mixture firmly and evenly into the dish. Place the baking dish in the refrigerator and let it chill for at least 2 hours, or until the bars have set.

Once the bars have set, use the parchment paper overhang to lift them out of the dish. Place the bars on a cutting board and use a sharp knife to cut them into squares or rectangles, depending on your preference.

INGREDIENTS:
- 1 cup dried figs
- 1 cup walnuts
- 1 cup old-fashioned oats
- 1/2 cup honey or maple syrup
- 1/4 cup creamy almond or peanut butter
- 1/2 teaspoon vanilla extract
- A pinch of salt (optional)

LEMON SORBET

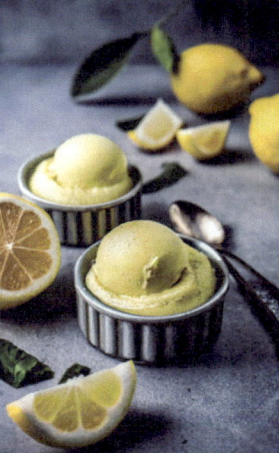

Start by preparing the lemons. Wash them thoroughly and zest the outer peel of 2-3 lemons. Set aside the zest. Cut the zested lemons in half and juice them. You'll need about 1 cup of fresh lemon juice. You can use a citrus juicer to extract the juice easily.

In a saucepan, combine granulated sugar and water. Place the saucepan over medium heat. Stir the sugar and water mixture until the sugar completely dissolves, creating a simple syrup. This should take about 3-5 minutes. Once the sugar has dissolved, remove the syrup from heat and let it cool.

Once the simple syrup has cooled, add the lemon zest and fresh lemon juice to it. Stir to combine, creating a lemon-flavored syrup. Pour the lemon syrup mixture into a shallow dish or a freezer-safe container. Ensure it's wide enough to allow for even freezing. Place the container in the freezer, uncovered.

After about an hour, check the sorbet. You'll notice that the edges start to freeze. Use a fork to scrape and mix the frozen edges into the liquid center. Repeat this process every 30 minutes for about 2-3 hours, or until the entire mixture has frozen into a sorbet consistency. This process helps create a smoother texture by preventing large ice crystals from forming. Once the Lemon Sorbet has reached the desired consistency, it's ready to serve.

- 4-5 large lemons (for juice and zest)
- 1 cup granulated sugar
- 1 cup water

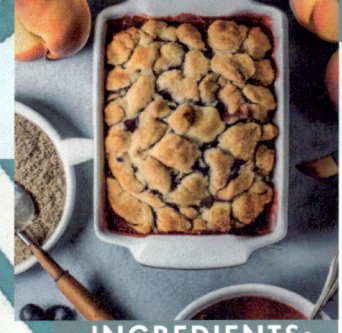

PEACH AND BERRY COBBLER

INGREDIENTS:
For the Filling:
- 2 cups sliced fresh or frozen peaches
- 1 cup mixed berries (your favorite variety)
- 1/4 cup granulated sugar
- 1 tbsp cornstarch
- 1/2 tsp vanilla extract (optional)

For the Cobbler Topping:
- 1 cup all-purpose flour
- 1/4 cup granulated sugar
- 1 1/2 tsp baking powder
- 1/2 tsp salt
- 1/2 cup unsalted butter
- 1/4 cup milk

COOKING PROCESS:
Preheat your oven to 350°F (175°C). Grease a baking dish or an ovenproof skillet.

For the Filling:
In a mixing bowl, combine: sliced fresh or thawed frozen peaches, mixed berries, granulated sugar (adjust the amount depending on the sweetness of the fruit), cornstarch, vanilla extract (if desired). Toss the fruit mixture gently to coat the fruit evenly with sugar and cornstarch. The cornstarch will help thicken the filling as it bakes.

Transfer the fruit mixture to the greased baking dish or skillet, spreading it out evenly.

For the Cobbler Topping:
In another mixing bowl, prepare combining: all-purpose flour, granulated sugar, baking powder, and salt (if desired). Add cold and cubed unsalted butter to the dry ingredients.

Use a pastry cutter or your fingers to cut the butter into the dry ingredients until the mixture resembles coarse crumbs. Pour in milk and stir until a thick, sticky dough forms.

Drop spoonfuls of the cobbler dough evenly over the fruit filling. You can leave some gaps for the fruit to peek through. Place the baking dish or skillet in the preheated oven and bake for approximately 35-40 minutes, or until the cobbler topping is golden brown and the fruit filling is bubbling.

Remove from the oven and let it cool slightly. Serve with a scoop of vanilla ice cream or a dollop of whipped cream.

BERRY AND YOGURT PARFAIT

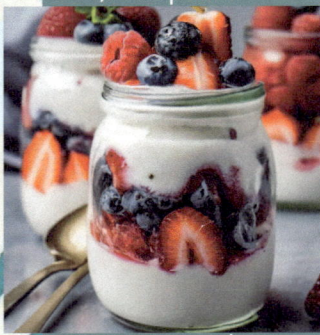

- 2 cups Greek yogurt (or your preferred yogurt)
- 1 cup mixed berries (your favorite variety)
- 1/2 cup granola
- 2 tablespoons honey (optional, for added sweetness)
- Fresh mint leaves for garnish

Start by preparing the berries. If using strawberries, hull and slice them into bite-sized pieces. Rinse all the berries and gently pat them dry with a paper towel.

In a separate bowl, mix the berries together to create a colorful and tasty berry medley. In individual serving glasses or bowls, begin assembling the parfaits.

Start with a layer of yogurt at the bottom of each glass. Use approximately 1/4 cup of yogurt for each serving. Add a layer of the mixed berries on top of the yogurt. Use about 1/4 cup of the berry medley for each serving.

Sprinkle 2 tbsp of granola over the berries. This adds a delightful crunch to the parfait. If you prefer a sweeter parfait, drizzle 1/2 tbsp of honey over the granola in each serving glass. Adjust the sweetness to your liking.

Repeat the layering process: yogurt, berries, granola, and honey (if desired) until you reach the top of the serving glasses. You can create as many layers as you like, depending on the size of your glasses.

Finish each parfait with a fresh mint leaf for a pop of color and added freshness.

Sweets to Savor Without Guilt

ORANGE AND DATE SALAD

COOKING PROCESS:

Start by preparing the oranges. Using a sharp knife, carefully slice off the top and bottom of each orange to create flat surfaces. This will make it easier to peel the oranges.

Stand the oranges upright on one of the flat ends and use your knife to carefully cut away the peel and pith, following the curve of the fruit. Make sure to remove all of the white pith as it can be bitter.

Once the oranges are peeled, hold them over a bowl to catch any juice, and slice them into thin rounds or segments. Collect any extra juice from the oranges in the bowl.

In a large serving bowl, combine the sliced oranges, chopped Medjool dates, and chopped fresh mint leaves. Gently toss the ingredients together to distribute them evenly. If you'd like to enhance the flavor, drizzle orange blossom water over the salad. This is optional and adds a fragrant citrusy note to the dish.

Optionally, drizzle a bit of honey over the salad for added sweetness, if desired. Adjust the sweetness to your preference. For a touch of warmth and spice, sprinkle a pinch of ground cinnamon over the salad. This is also optional and complements the sweetness of the dates and oranges.

Gently toss the salad again to coat the ingredients with the optional additions. To serve, divide the Orange and Date Salad into four individual serving dishes or plates. If you like, garnish each serving with a sprinkle of crushed pistachios for added texture and a nutty flavor.

INGREDIENTS:
- 4 large navel oranges
- 8-10 Medjool dates
- 1/4 cup chopped fresh mint leaves
- 2 tbsp orange blossom water (optional)
- A drizzle of honey
- A pinch of cinnamon
- Crushed pistachios for garnish (optional)

COCONUT CHIA PUDDING

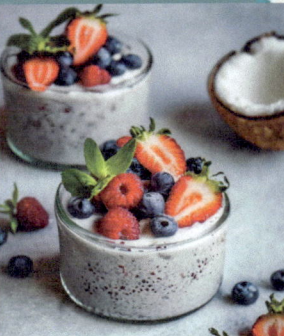

In a mixing bowl, combine chia seeds, and coconut milk (you can use full-fat coconut milk for a creamier texture or lite coconut milk for a lighter option). Add maple syrup or honey to the mixture. Adjust the sweetness to your liking. You can add more or less depending on your preference.

Optionally, add vanilla extract for a hint of flavor. Stir everything together thoroughly. Once the ingredients are well combined, cover the mixing bowl and refrigerate it for at least 4 hours or overnight. This allows the chia seeds to absorb the liquid and create a pudding-like consistency.

After the resting period, give the mixture a good stir to ensure that the chia seeds are evenly distributed. Divide the Pudding into dishes or glasses. If desired, top each serving with fresh fruit, berries, or nuts. Sliced strawberries, blueberries, or shredded coconut are popular choices for garnish.

- 1/2 cup chia seeds
- 2 cups coconut milk (full-fat or lite)
- 2 tablespoons maple syrup or honey (adjust to taste)
- 1/2 teaspoon vanilla extract (optional)
- Fresh fruit, berries, or nuts for topping (optional)

Sweets to Savor Without Guilt

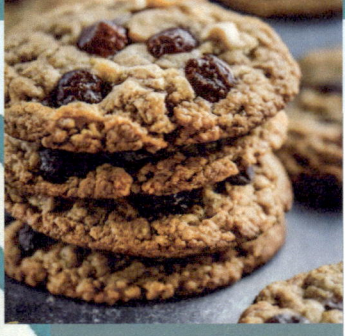

OATMEAL RAISIN COOKIES

COOKING PROCESS:

Preheat your oven to 350°F (175°C). Line a baking sheet with parchment paper or lightly grease it to prevent sticking.
In a mixing bowl, combine old-fashioned oats, all-purpose flour, baking soda, ground cinnamon, and a pinch of salt (if desired). Stir the dry ingredients together until well combined and set them aside.
In another mixing bowl, cream together: softened unsalted butter, brown sugar, and granulated sugar. Add egg and vanilla extract and mix until the wet ingredients are well combined and the mixture becomes creamy. Gradually add the dry ingredient mixture to the wet ingredients. Mix until all the ingredients are fully incorporated and form a cookie dough. Fold in raisins (or more if you prefer a generous amount of raisins). The raisins add natural sweetness and a chewy texture.
Drop rounded tbsp of cookie dough onto the prepared baking sheet, spacing them about 2 inches apart to allow room for spreading during baking. Use the back of a fork to gently flatten each cookie and create a crisscross pattern on top. Bake in the preheated oven for approximately 10-12 minutes, or until the cookies are golden brown around the edges.
Remove the cookies from the oven and let them cool on the baking sheet for a few minutes to set. After cooling slightly, transfer the Cookies to a wire rack to cool completely.

INGREDIENTS:

- 1 cup old-fashioned oats
- 1/2 cup all-purpose flour
- 1/2 tsp baking soda
- 1/2 tsp ground cinnamon
- A pinch of salt (optional)
- 1/2 cup unsalted butter
- 1/2 cup brown sugar
- 1/4 cup granulated sugar
- 1 large egg
- 1 tsp vanilla extract
- 1/2 cup raisins (or more to taste)

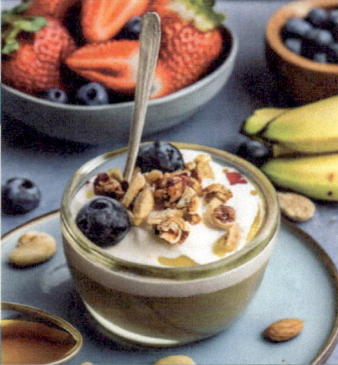

BANANA "NICE" CREAM

Start by peeling the ripe bananas and slicing them into coins. It's a good idea to slice them into small pieces for easier blending. Place the banana slices in a single layer on a baking sheet lined with parchment paper. Freeze the banana slices for at least 2-3 hours, or until they are completely frozen. This step is crucial for achieving the creamy texture of "nice" cream.
Once the banana slices are frozen, remove them from the freezer. Add the frozen banana slices to a food processor or a high-speed blender. If desired, add 1 teaspoon of vanilla extract for extra flavor.
Blend the banana slices until they become smooth and creamy. You may need to stop and scrape down the sides of the processor or blender a few times to ensure even blending.
The texture should resemble that of soft-serve ice cream. If it's too thick, you can add a small amount of milk (dairy or plant-based) to help with blending, but be cautious not to add too much.
Once you have achieved a creamy consistency, scoop the cream into serving bowls or glasses. Now comes the fun part! Customize your cream with toppings of your choice. Fresh berries, chopped nuts, and a drizzle of honey are all excellent options.

- 4 ripe bananas
- 1 tsp vanilla extract (optional)
- Toppings of your choice, such as fresh berries, nuts, or a drizzle of honey

Sweets to Savor Without Guilt

ROASTED FRUIT SALAD

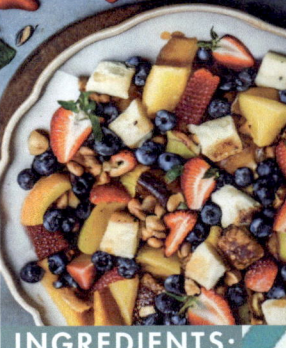

COOKING PROCESS:

Preheat your oven to 375°F (190°C).
Wash, peel (if necessary), and chop the fruits into bite-sized pieces. You can use a combination of fruits like strawberries, pineapple, peaches, or any fruits that you enjoy. The choice is flexible and can vary based on what's in season.
In a large mixing bowl, combine the chopped fruits. Drizzle honey or maple syrup over the fruits. Adjust the sweetness to your liking.
Sprinkle cinnamon over the fruits for a warm and aromatic flavor. If you prefer, you can add a pinch of salt to enhance the taste, but this is optional. Gently toss the fruits to ensure they are well coated with the honey (or maple syrup) and cinnamon mixture.
Transfer the coated fruits to a baking dish or a baking sheet lined with parchment paper. Spread them out in an even layer.
Roast the fruits in the preheated oven for approximately 15-20 minutes, or until they become slightly caramelized and tender.
The exact roasting time may vary depending on the fruits you use, so keep an eye on them to prevent overcooking.
Once roasted, remove the fruits from the oven and let them cool slightly.
You can serve the Roasted Fruit Salad warm as a dessert or a side dish, or you can let it cool completely and serve it chilled.
For an extra touch, serve the roasted fruits with a dollop of Greek yogurt or vanilla yogurt for a delightful contrast of flavors and textures.
Optionally, garnish the dish with fresh mint leaves for a burst of freshness and visual appeal.

INGREDIENTS:
- 4 cups mixed fruits (fruit of your choice)
- 2 tablespoons honey or maple syrup
- 1 teaspoon cinnamon
- A pinch of salt (optional)
- Greek yogurt or vanilla yogurt for serving (optional)
- Fresh mint leaves for garnish (optional)

PAPAYA WITH LIME

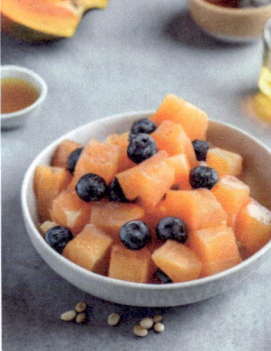

Begin by selecting ripe papaya. A ripe papaya should have vibrant orange flesh and yield slightly to gentle pressure when touched.
Cut the papaya in half lengthwise. Use a spoon to scoop out and discard the seeds from the center of the papaya halves. Slice the papaya flesh into bite-sized cubes or slices. You can be creative with the shapes you prefer.
Place the cubed or sliced papaya in a serving bowl.
Cut the limes in half, and squeeze the juice from all four halves over the papaya. The lime juice adds a zesty and tangy flavor that complements the sweetness of the papaya.
Drizzle honey or maple syrup over the papaya. Adjust the sweetness to your liking, as the amount of sweetener needed may vary depending on the ripeness of the papaya. Gently toss the papaya, lime juice, and sweetener together to ensure the flavors are evenly distributed.
Let the Papaya with Lime sit for a few minutes to allow the flavors to meld together. Optionally, garnish the dish with fresh mint leaves for added freshness and visual appeal.

- 1 ripe papaya
- 2 limes
- 2 tablespoons honey or maple syrup
- Fresh mint leaves for garnish (optional)

Sweets to Savor Without Guilt

ALPHABETICAL RECIPE INDEX

ALMOND AND HONEY RICE PUDDING..................14
ALMOND DATE BALLS..................7
AVOCADO AND BLACK BEAN SALSA..................5
BAKED APPLES WITH CINNAMON..................68
BAKED HALIBUT WITH TOMATOES AND OLIVES..................55
BAKED SALMON WITH LEMON AND DILL..................55
BANANA "NICE" CREAM..................72
BANANA WALNUT MUFFINS..................13
BARLEY AND MUSHROOM SOUP..................17
BERRY AND YOGURT PARFAIT..................70
BIFTEKIA (GRILLED MEAT PATTIES)..................64
BLUEBERRY OATMEAL BARS..................8
BROWN RICE AND BLACK BEAN BOWL..................54
CABBAGE AND CARROT SLAW..................32
CABBAGE AND POTATO SOUP..................19
CAPRESE SALAD..................30
CAPRESE SKEWERS..................62
CHIA SEED PUDDING..................7
CLASSIC HUMMUS..................9
COCONUT CHIA PUDDING..................71
CUCUMBER CUPS WITH TUNA SALAD..................30
DATE AND NUT ENERGY BITES..................6
DATE AND NUT STUFFED BAKED APPLES..................12
DELICIOUS WHOLE WHEAT PITA BREAD..................36
EASY TERIYAKI SALMON..................58
EGGPLANT AND TOMATO BRUSCHETTA..................11
EGGPLANT AND WALNUT ROLLS..................64
EGGPLANT AND ZUCCHINI RATATOUILLE..................67
EXOTIC MISO-GLAZED SALMON..................59
FALAFEL WITH HUMMUS AND BULGUR SALAD..................60
FIG AND WALNUT BARS..................69
FLAVORFUL LEMON AND GARLIC ROASTED CHICKEN..................47
GREEN PEA AND MINT SOUP..................24
GRILLED CHICKEN WITH HERBED QUINOA..................48
GRILLED EGGPLANT AND ZUCCHINI RATATOUILLE..................53
GRILLED OCTOPUS..................56
GRILLED WHOLE SEA BASS..................58
HUMMUS MEZZE PLATTE..................8
KALE AND WHITE BEAN SOUP..................16
LEMON SORBET..................69
LENTIL AND VEGETABLE SOUP..................15
LENTIL AND VEGETABLE STEW..................40
MEDITERRANEAN BAKED EGGPLANT PARMESAN..................66
MEDITERRANEAN CHICKPEA SALAD..................28
MEDITERRANEAN HERB AND OLIVE HUMMUS..................10
MEDITERRANEAN ROASTED EGGPLANT..................40

MEDITERRANEAN STUFFED GRAPE LEAVES	61
MEDITERRANEAN TABBOULEH SALAD	31
MEDITERRANEAN WHOLE GRAIN BREAD	34
MINESTRONE SOUP	27
MISO SOUP WITH TOFU AND SEAWEED	26
OATMEAL RAISIN COOKIES	72
OKINAWAN BRAISED PORK BELLY	62
OKINAWAN SEARED AHI TUNA SALAD	29
OKINAWAN SEARED TUNA STEAK	56
OKINAWAN STIR-FRIED VEGETABLES	47
OKINAWAN SWEET POTATO BREAD	36
OKINAWAN TOFU AND SEAWEED SALAD	32
ORANGE AND DATE SALAD	71
OSSO BUCO (VEAL OR BEEF SHANK STEW)	49
PAPAYA WITH LIME	73
PEACH AND BERRY COBBLER	70
QUINOA AND BLACK BEAN STUFFED PEPPERS	45
QUINOA AND VEGETABLE SOUP	22
QUINOA-STUFFED BELL PEPPERS	51
REGIONAL MOCHI BREAD	37
ROASTED ASPARAGUS WITH LEMON AND PARMESAN	38
ROASTED BEET AND GOAT CHEESE CROSTINI	41
ROASTED FRUIT SALAD	73
ROASTED GARLIC AND WHITE BEAN DIP	50
ROASTED RED PEPPER AND WALNUT DIP	42
SARDINIAN FREGOLA WITH CLAMS	57
SARDINIAN LAMB AND ARTICHOKE STEW	63
SARDINIAN PANE CARASAU (FLATBREAD)	35
SAUTÉED GREENS WITH WHITE BEANS	54
SPANAKOPITA (SPINACH PIE)	65
SPINACH AND CHICKPEA SOUP	18
SPINACH AND FETA STUFFED MINI PEPPERS	43
STUFFED MUSHROOMS WITH QUINOA AND SPINACH	43
SUNNY CAPRESE STUFFED PORTOBELLO MUSHROOMS	44
SWEET POTATO AND CHICKPEA PATTIES	39
SWEET POTATO AND GINGER SOUP	21
TASTY SALAD WITH GRILLED CHICKEN	33
TOFU AND VEGETABLE STIR-FRY	52
TOMATO LENTIL SOUP	20
TURMERIC AND CAULIFLOWER SOUP	23
TZATZIKI CUCUMBER SALAD	28
VEGAN MISO SOUP	25
VEGAN TAGINE WITH CHICKPEAS	46
VIBRANT SUSHI BOWLS	57
WALNUT-STUFFED DATES	6
WATERMELON AND FETA SKEWERS	5
WHOLE WHEAT PASTA PRIMAVERA	53
WHOLESOME TZATZIKI AND VEGGIE PLATTER	41
ZUCCHINI AND TOMATO SKEWERS	51

Embrace Plant-Based Wonders:
Incorporate more plant-based ingredients into your meals. These nutrient-packed wonders not only enhance flavor but also contribute to overall well-being.

Savor Mindfully, Eat Joyfully:
Practice mindful eating. Take the time to savor each bite, appreciating the textures and flavors. Eating joyfully is not just about nourishing the body but also nurturing the soul.

Connect Through Cooking:
Cooking is not just a chore; it's an opportunity to connect with the ingredients and the people around you. Share the joy of cooking with loved ones; it's a bond that transcends generations.

Prioritize Quality Over Quantity:
Choose quality ingredients over quantity. It's not about how much you eat but the quality of what you consume that truly matters.

Stay Active, Stay Alive:
Incorporate movement into your daily routine. Whether it's a brisk walk, a dance session, or a yoga class, staying active is a key ingredient for a vibrant life.

May these tips accompany you on your culinary and wellness journey. Here's to a life filled with delectable flavors, shared moments, and the timeless wisdom of savoring every bite.

Closing this chapter on the recipes from the Blue Zones, I realize these pages only scratch the surface of a rich culinary tapestry. They mark merely the beginning of our exploration and tasting journey through the flavors and traditions of the Blue Zones.

This book serves as an introduction, a tantalizing glimpse into the world of longevity and taste intertwined. It lays the foundation for a deeper understanding of how food shapes our lives, drawing from cultures where health and vitality are celebrated through what we eat.

However, as we bid adieu to this collection, I'm thrilled to announce our next culinary expedition—an exploration of the stunning island of Sardinia. Known for its breathtaking beaches, this island is not only a paradise for the eyes but a treasure trove of gastronomic wonders waiting to be discovered.

In the upcoming book, we'll traverse the landscapes of Sardinia's cuisine, uncovering the secrets behind its iconic dishes and traditions. Prepare to immerse yourself in a world where history, culture, and taste converge to create an unparalleled culinary experience.

Manufactured by Amazon.ca
Bolton, ON